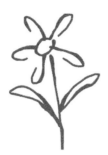

Grow Through
What You Go Through

Facing Mental Health Struggles

Grow Through What You Go Through

How to Plant Seeds for Personal Growth

By Jill VanderZanden

Growth Flower Publishing

Grow Through What You Go Through:
How to Plant Seeds for Personal Growth
written by: Jill (VanderZanden) Bilka
www.JillWithaFlower.com

First Edition, Published by: Growth Flower Publishing

P.O Box 364 - Dundee, OR 97115
GrowthFlowerPublishing@gmail.com

ISBN 979-8-9859285-0-1 (eBook), ISBN 979-8-9859285-1-8 (paperback)
Library of Congress Control Number: 2022910061
Printed in the United States. Amazon KDP Print on Demand Services. If there are errors with printing or binding, please contact Amazon Support.

This book is not a substitute for the advice of a mental health or medical professional.

Dedication

For My Dad - he taught me how to be a hard worker, to live with integrity, to help my community, to love with fierce gentleness, that family comes first, and if you want something done right, do it yourself. I wouldn't tenacious beer loving girl I am without him!

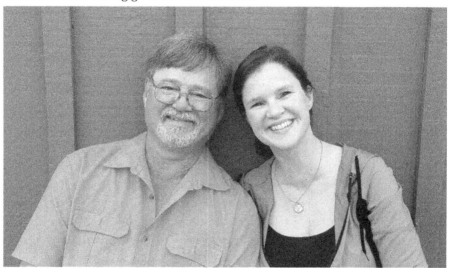

My dad passed away when I was in the middle of drafting this book, and I chose to publish with my maiden name in his honor. As the youngest of three girls, this is one way to continue my family name. In his last days, I reassured him that he raised me to be strong as I knew he was worried about me with it being so recent that I found out my mental health diagnosis. I told him that he could be at peace and know I would be okay. I promised I'd take real good care of myself and that he didn't have to worry about me. When he passed just days later, I knew I would keep that promise.

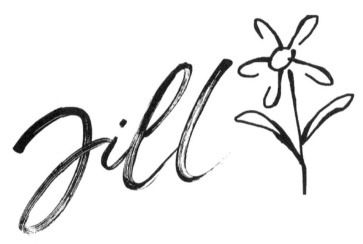

As a child, before I could read and identify my own name, at social events my parents would write my name on a cup and put a flower at the end, so I knew it was mine. As I got a bit older and started to write my own name, I would still write it with a flower on occasion. Although I'm all grown up now and know how to spell my name without a flower, it has stuck with me throughout my life. Some people have spirit animals, but I've always been more of a flower kind of girl. I am forever thankful for the roots of my family and larger community which enriched who I have grown to be.

Flowers have continued to be a symbol of growth in my professional endeavors as well as my personal journey to wellness, and now here as my writing blooms. Unlike the weather, we have our own seasons and time to bloom. Growth is the evidence of life and often the seed is the moment we accept our own weaknesses and choose to do the work to change and reach for a brighter version of life. May we all bloom where we are planted and remember that everything grows with love.

Growth Tool

You'll see this flower symbol Growth Tool **as you turn the pages to help you find tips and tools more easily throughout the book.**

Table of Contents

*Resources included at end of book

Preface

Let me tell you a story of how this book came to be written. Looking back, I can appreciate a few good things came from this wild chapter in my life. But in reality, it was a bit of a nightmare. It was an enlightenment on the struggles of humanity if you will. It was a month in my life I will forever remember.

At the end of February 2021, the week I started relationship counseling, my husband noticed I had a big patch of hair loss on the back of my head. My mind went to the darkest places since I knew I had also been experiencing some confusing thoughts and feelings I couldn't explain. Something happened that altered the state of my being and put my mind into overdrive. I thought perhaps I was some magical mix of Wonder Woman and a Disney princess that could help save the world. I was certain if I wrote and shared the right words or sang like a Disney princess, I was going to heal everyone. All the hurt in the world. I was inspired in so many ways and became a supercharged cheerleader of life. While worrying about my health and relationship, I started to write out the bursts of thoughts and feelings I was having. A few hours later, having typed several thousand words, my mind recalled the movies *A Beautiful Mind* and *Phenomenon* and I was sure I must be dying or having some psychotic break.

Between the pandemic reality of distance learning my three kids, working from home, and failing at managing life in general, I wrote the first approximately 26,500 words of this book in seven days. I was sure I had a brain tumor. In my mind, it was the only answer that added up. I was barely eating, drinking, or sleeping. All I could focus on was writing down the inspired thoughts in my brain. I figured if I was going to die, I might as well leave some instructions and inspiration to guide those I left behind. That is how this book was born, and over the next year, this baby grew.

Let me rewind a bit further to the Fall of 2020. I created a group through social media called "Positive Thinking, Community & Support." My goal was to connect like-minded people who were struggling with negativity whether in their own thoughts, their homes, or the social climate and uncertainty outside their door. It was a time where many felt isolated and disconnected from their regular communities and support networks. So, in creating this group I was offering an opportunity for connection and a place where people could share their struggles, successes, or simply tools for support. I shared resources and words of encouragement about self-care, growth mindset, wellness, empathy, progress over perfection, compassionate communication, creating healthy habits, building relationships, and other topics to work toward a healthier and happier version of ourselves. I shared many moments of vulnerability and personal struggle alongside encouraging words, resources, and images in the months leading up to what I now call my mental health or midlife awakening. By writing and sharing with the hopes of helping others, I was saving myself. Sure, the group grew little by little and what I was writing had resonated with the group. When I looked back at what I had shared, I realized I had created a playbook—my own personal recipe to wellness. Or at least a really good start.

I began to write as a way of processing my thoughts and feelings. By letting them flow, I released the hard I was facing and troubleshot ways to fix the broken parts. Now, a year later, I find myself referencing the words I have shared in this book to help me through hard days. On days when I feel myself drowning in hard, I look back to days I shared strength and remember that I can pick myself up again if I simply do what I've encouraged others to do. We all need reminders from time to time about how to continue down a good and healthy path. Despite it being one of the darkest and hardest times in my life, filled with unexpected life changes, loss, and uncertainty, I found a bright perspective. I am an optimist and believe we can't stop looking for silver linings and moments of gratitude, even in tough times.

As of this writing, it's been a year now since my brain went into overdrive. I am back to my regular self, out of crisis mode, and know I am not a mix of Wonder Woman, Elsa, and Little Mermaid. I do not have magical powers and was not put on Earth to save anyone. Though in my heightened state, I do think I had a few enlightening thoughts as I was able to think with confidence *in* myself. I was not crushed by all the self-doubt and fear I usually lived with. Perhaps some of the thoughts I share from before my brain crashed will resonate with you and help you develop questions to get your thinker thinking. It clearly got mine going.

Once I was well, and luckily not dying, I came back, edited, and added more words to the mix. It's still amazing to think much of this book came from out of the perfect storm of crisis—one very intense week that ended in a crash and the diagnosis of a mental health condition. As I moved toward the big 4-

0, I continued to focus on my wellness. I chose to sign up for my first organized run, a "Bee Kind" 5K, and got friends to join me and marked other things off my bucket list. In life, you can look at your time and experiences as filled with obstacles, or you can see the opportunities. I prefer the latter.

Introduction

There I stood at a major intersection less than a mile from my house. I was barefoot, broken, and confused after crashing into another vehicle and sending it across the highway. The morning leading up to the crash was a bit of a blur. I had been frantically writing, up since about 3:00 am, which was the trend for over a week now. I was trying to capture all the inspired thoughts I was having. My husband and I had gotten into an argument about my fixation on writing and I had this urgent sense I needed to leave the house. I grabbed my keys and ran from my house barefoot, in my pajamas, hair unbrushed, no make-up, and without any identification. Once on the road, I got this frightening feeling a friend was in imminent danger. So, I hit the gas to hurriedly drive to their house in hopes I could get there in time to save them. In this altered state, nothing was going to stop me. Until I crashed.

I got out of my car, amazingly unharmed, and began to run towards my friend's house. Emergency responders stopped me from running into the highway and at that moment, I thought they were stopping me from saving my friend. I got back in my vehicle afraid and locked the doors. I remember an officer pounding on the window and yelling at me. I was afraid and didn't want to get out. I felt I was in danger. I don't remember how I got out of my vehicle. Next thing I remember is being pushed against my car with force, my arms being pulled behind my back in such a way I was crying and sure my arms might break. A police officer was putting handcuffs on me, and I didn't understand why. I was screaming for help, screaming for the emergency responders to listen to me, and screaming for them to pray with me. I only remember screaming. I was still worried for my friend and wanted emergency responders to go to his house to help the family. Next thing I know they were putting me on a gurney and cutting my sweatshirt to give me some sort of shot and loading me into an ambulance. I was crying and afraid and don't remember another thing until I was in an emergency room. I continued to feel as though someone was trying to hurt me. I felt I was in danger.

I was not myself; I was terrified and confused, and not fully in control of my actions. It was the beginning of the most terrifying and difficult weeks of my life, and the first and hopefully only time I'd be in cuffs. The experience with the police left me bruised, not just physically but mentally.

In the ER, my husband was beside me the whole time trying to comfort me and respond to the many people who were worried about me. I didn't trust him. I had fled the house not only to save my friend, but because I thought I was in danger in my own home. I had hit the wall of feeling able to manage all the stress in my life and went into fight and flight mode. The hospital staff together with the emergency responders deduced that I was having a mental health crisis. You see, our brains are much like a computer, and mine overheated, crashed, and needed a reboot. From the emergency room, I was transported in the night to a mental health hospital for assessment and treatment where I spent the next two weeks. Physically I was fine, but I needed help and medications to get my mental health back in good shape and return me to being me again.

Like any good gossip, those closest to me noticed the warning signs of trouble before I saw it myself. My family tried to have an intervention as they worried I was sharing too many personal things on Facebook. Some friends mentioned they were concerned I was losing too much weight. Others were questioning if I was seeking support from the wrong people or in the wrong places. It wasn't until after I was home from the hospital that I learned just how many people had been talking about me and my recent behavior with concern. I know it was with caring. but it was still hard to know I was the center of attention and in the spotlight under less than favorable circumstances. At first, I felt ashamed and embarrassed that I needed help to get back to a healthy version of me. Then, I began to realize we all have a messy or wild chapter, and through those challenging times, we also have the opportunity to learn and grow. For anyone who may be struggling or has gone through a challenging time, know you are not alone. Reaching out for counseling, treatment of some kind, or trying medications to help is okay. We all have times when we're in need of a little help— sometimes in big ways. Despite the mess I'd caused, my husband supported me and helped extinguish the fires I inadvertently started.

I hope some of the things I learned from my breakdown help you have a breakthrough, too, and support you on your path to wellness. I hope you'll discover things about yourself and truths within your heart that will lead you where you need to go next. Life is one big learning lesson, and I hope the words I share help you reflect on yours. May you choose to see the hope and possibilities of what life can be. From each struggle in life we can learn, grow, and find true happiness and success. This isn't just my story, it's a story of all the people who have touched my life and shared their insight, experience, and perspectives. The world may feel big, but we each play a significant role in the lives of the people in our little corner of it.

I am passionate about communication and words and appreciate we all see life differently. I hope you'll open your mind and heart to see it through my eyes as you read these pages. Whether you agree or disagree with the words that follow, hopefully, they will encourage you to think about what truly matters in your life. I'm here to encourage you there's more to your story, and to share with you a bit of mine. There are no shortcuts to growth and success. A happier, healthier life is all about choices. Better days are ahead of us if we believe in the power to change, for the good. One day at a time, with the right perspective and choosing the next right, helpful action!

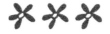

words to grow by

"Life is ten percent what happens to you and ninety percent how you respond to it."

Charles Swindoll

"The best way to predict your future is to create it."

Abraham Lincoln

"It's never too late – never too late to start over, never too late to be happy."

Jane Fonda

"Never let the fear of striking out keep you from playing the game."

Babe Ruth

"When one door closes, another opens; but we often look so long and so regretfully upon the closed door that we do not see the one that has opened for us."

Alexander Graham Bell

Chapter 1
A Path to Personal Growth

More people than we realize are hitting a wall, trying to fake it 'til they make it. The new term I like to use is "Be Real While You Heal." Now don't take this to mean everyone has big trauma to heal from. Some do, for sure. But what can sneak up on us are the little traumas that, over time, manifest in our lives in big ways. From the minute memories and experiences of childhood to the interactions and insecurities built in adolescence and the patterns and communication breakdowns that are further solidified through our adult relationships. We all have some level of brokenness to heal from. Even those that appear to have the "perfect lives" are plagued by imperfections that weigh life down. This heaviness that we carry causes an unnecessary burden. By recognizing this weight, we can allow ourselves to heal and understand that with some effort we can ease the burden that weighs life down. There is so often room for improvement boiling under the surface. The first step is to stop pretending. To feign strength when we experience weaknesses does not build a strong foundation for growth and happiness. Improvement starts within, that is where our only control lies.

When we are stuck in a loop that is not fulfilling or bringing us joy, it can be a sign that we need to shake things up. Every day we should have a goal, at least one little thing, to remind us about what we are passionate about. When we slow down, rid of distractions, open our minds, think with our heart, and get a little inspiration from a higher spirit or energy—we open the door to new possibilities. During the coronavirus pandemic that came crashing down on our world in 2020, and continued for more than two years, I hit a wall of feeling out of control. Many others found similar challenges from the added stress and pressure.

Out of my breakdown, I learned to embrace that spark and vision that spoke to my heart instead of doing what I had done in the past. My old habits were no longer working. I call that spark *passion*. I discovered the mountain I was meant to climb in life. Let's call that *purpose*. I started envisioning the steps and actions I needed to take to get to my dream destination. I'll call that my *path*.

This was the high point of this treacherous time. I wasn't sure where my inspired passion and purpose were leading, but I was unknowingly making a path to get there. I was creating my plan for personal growth. With a background in psychology, communication, teaching, social work, and community building, I have always carried a desire to care for and help others. So, I continued to type feverishly like a kid in a candy store, so excited for any sweetness I could share with others. As such, this book is full of heartfelt words, thoughtful tools, and specific action steps for personal growth, and I wrap it all up with a little inspiration and encouragement. I hope this work resonates with you and helps you discover what matters in your life and your next steps.

Passion & Purpose

To work towards personal growth, it's helpful to know what you're passionate about. What do you genuinely care about? What drives you? What inspires you to act? What makes you feel happy? We all care about different things, but we all care about something. Without care in the world, apathy develops. If you haven't considered it in a while, if you've been going through the motions of life without purpose—you are not alone. At some point, everyone reaches a grey area in life. A time when we struggle to remember what we like, what we're good at, or who we are. Those moments, days, months, or years are hard. Once you recognize you are in that grey area, start turning back the pages, peeling back the layers, and finding the beautiful colors that make your heart whole. Happiness lives within us, but sometimes we have to dig deeper to find it.

So, how do move through and forward from that grey area? By using it as an opportunity to pause and take time to listen to your heart and what is at the core of who you are and who you want to be. When you leave this Earth, how will people remember you? No, it's not about being famous or world-known—it's about the positive impact you can make in your circle. What difference will you make for yourself, within your family, or in the lives of your friends, your neighbors, and your community? In your most direct circle of impact, how are you engaged and showing up? Are you a positive addition, acting in the ways you'd want to be remembered? A way that makes a difference not only for yourself but for those around you? By discovering your passion and sharing it with others, you will make a difference in life, you will help something or someone to be better. That's what happens when you care and care enough to act. One person can make a difference! Some days it may feel like a crawl and others a sprint. As long as you're headed in the right direction, just keep your chin up and your eyes forward. We may not know exactly what tomorrow will bring, but we can hold our heads high, think positive, and expect the best.

We only live once, and I'm not here for the small talk. My story is here to help you see things in a different light and to challenge you to be the best version of yourself. In case you haven't had people cheering for you to succeed, I am here to cheer you on. **You can be successful and achieve anything you put your mind to when you believe it in your heart.** I am so excited to see you realize that for yourself! I know it is possible, and I want to help you climb that mountain one step at a time. Every human is intrinsically good and has the potential to do remarkable things. Sometimes that good is buried under years of trauma, lack of support, love, or confidence. Once you realize what's holding you back, there will be nothing to stop you from moving forward. That's an exciting thought, isn't it? There is no better day than today to discover the happiest day of your life.

Do you want to help make changes in yourself and others? Believing that responsibility falls solely on your shoulders can be overwhelming. It starts with all of us taking small actions. It takes the unique strengths of each of us to make the biggest things happen. So, let's work together and move up this mountain, shall we? With each new year, new month, new day, or new hour that passes in our life, we can make a new choice. Will you choose to go through life on autopilot, or will you choose to stand out? Don't be afraid to show your true colors and chase your dreams.

To live a version of life that makes you succeed and smile, you need to be willing to grow and work towards it. Are you settling for less because it seems easier? Are you stepping back from opportunities for fear of failing? Step away from that fear and be confident in the fact you get what you work for in life. Find your passion and purpose and follow it! Get on your path to happiness. I am cheering for you to reach that next step. Good things rarely happen overnight, so don't give up!

For too long now some of us have been putting pressure on ourselves to carry or maintain the happiness of others. For those who did not inherit a people-pleasing gene, I want to high five you right now—I am so glad you never carried that weight. For others, like myself, I challenge you to release that burden. It is a burden none of us can carry for long. We can add to people's happiness, but they control the foundation of their feelings. Our recipe for true happiness lives inside, and it is important to recognize this and not assume we'll attain it from an external source.

Baking Up Your Own Recipe for Happiness

Let me explain this in a tasty way to help it make sense: Everybody is responsible for baking their own cake. We are responsible for discovering the core of our happiness in life, just as everyone else is responsible for discovering theirs. We are a part of the lives of others to add a little layer of frosting or some sprinkles on top. We are all intrinsically able to add sweetness to the life of others. But the secret to baking a sweet cake is to have fewer cooks in the kitchen. Everyone has their magic recipe and for too long we've been stirring things up, and not in a good way. So, let's take a step back from assuming we know the secret or can control anyone else's happiness. We need to consider ourselves the sprinkles, not the entire cake. So, let's start by focusing on our own recipe and what we can bake up in our own lives. Perhaps you're reading this and thinking, sounds great, but I have no sense of my passions.

Growth
Tool

Rediscovering Your Passion

If you've been stuck in a loop of day-to-day living and feeling unfulfilled, how do you change? How do you find your recipe for happiness?

Here are 10 things to help you find that spark:

- Reflect on your life and think of things you've excelled at or done well.

- What do your friends or peers consider you good or skilled at?

- What did you want to be when you were a kid and how does that compare to what you're doing now?

- Make a list of things or experiences that bring you joy. Which of these would you like to do more of?

- Consider what impact you want to make in the world or what would you like to be known for?

- Perhaps you need a fresh perspective. Why not sign up for a class to learn something new?

- If you haven't delved into community activities, now is a wonderful time to start!

- Read books, listen to podcasts, or find articles on topics that engage your inner spark. Topics that excite, inspire, and motivate you to take action and make positive changes.

- Create a vision board. Sometimes visuals can help you build a clearer picture of your goals or where you want to go next.

- Make time for activities, people, and places that bring you joy and excitement—get out of the mundane loops of life.

Ultimately it comes down to figuring out what it is you are doing when the little voice inside you says, "This, this right here is why I am here." A little flicker in your heart grows and you feel a warm glow because you know it's true. When that happens, pause, enjoy the moment, and allow more moments like that to occur.

My Pandemic Perspective

Can I tell you what I learned during the Pandemic, what my silver lining was? I realized it wasn't a time to clean house, which, don't tell anyone, but I never jumped on that bandwagon. No. Instead, I embraced the mess. I may have cleaned up for a couple of days, but I quickly realized as the mother of a family of five that I couldn't control that part of life and attempting to would not bring me joy. Instead, I chose to focus on decluttering my life of the noise, people, things, experiences, past hurt, and priorities that no longer served me. We are all on a different path. Perhaps you feel you are at a crossroads of choices that feel impossible to make due to the fear that you don't know what is coming next. At times we must move forward blindly, and trust that our choices, intentions, and actions will lead us to where we need to be.

During the pandemic, I went through the most uncertain and hardest year of my life being stretched and pushed in ways I never expected. My experience was like many others, yet unique as it was through my eyes and perspective. As a work-at-home mother who had transitioned into the first year of all my kids being in school, I had that bit of independence taken away as they all came back home for distance learning. Of course, it wasn't what they wanted either, so it was a constant battle of helping them understand I was temporarily wearing the new hat of teacher and wanted to help them be successful in this new setting. It began as a constant battle of screen rage as we were not a huge fan of personal electronic devices before the pandemic, and remote learning was almost all online. As a self-employed businesswoman with my own home office set up a decade earlier, I now had to share my office with my husband who was required to work from home. With him at home, my work became a back seat priority. I went back to working nights as I was now expected to teach my children during the day. While he was working at home, I had to manage the house in a new way as he often was on calls, so the noise level and distractions had to be kept at bay. Ever been in a house with three boys and tried to keep them quiet? Perhaps that was why my hair began to fall out!

As a woman, I felt overwhelmed managing these new stressors on top of the full plate I was already balancing. As a wife, I felt unseen, unvalued, and alone as I muddled through it all by myself as I felt our support and communication styles did not align. As a mother, I felt like a failure as my kids struggled with school and my house felt like it was becoming a negative and toxic war zone. The extrovert part of me felt so isolated from my community which had always been my outlet. As an optimist, I felt I had to stay afloat with a smile so as not to add to the weight of anyone else's hardships. The empathetic part of me felt the weight of all the conflict, fear, sadness, loss, and other hard feelings those around me were experiencing. Once again that awful people pleaser trait came out to play and took on the responsibility of trying to keep everyone happy. A task that, given the circumstances, was impossible. With my psychology background, I was seeing all the mental health effects of this tumultuous time and felt helpless in being able to fix any of it. These pandemic stressors added to the ordinary life challenges we'd already confronted. After a year of this, the implosion hit—a breakdown crashed upon me.

Until you have lived through a mournful time, it's hard to appreciate the brighter times as fully. We all have wild and messy lives—it's called being human. I am not writing because I know it all, nor am I telling you how to live your life. I am writing my story to impart the lessons I've learned. The moment we quit learning, growing, and striving for more is the moment we settle. We can all learn from and with each other as we strive for a better tomorrow. I have learned that living a wholesome life with a focus on balance and wellness is a big part of creating a better tomorrow.

Yes, there will continue to be negative, sad, and bad things happening in the world. We can't control those things. It's important to focus on the good and keep moving forward with the next right and helpful action we can take to make a difference in our life as well as in the families, businesses, and communities that surround us. To make big changes we must start small. We have the power to impact and improve life for ourselves and those around us. Open your heart and mind to listen and allow yourself to be led by your beliefs and passions. The power has always been inside you to make your dreams come true, so listen to those whispers of intuition, look for the signs, and hear the messages.

How does one listen to whispers of intuition? Some may call it paying attention to your gut, but that makes me think of my stomach growling. That thought makes me hungry, which I guess is a great time to listen to your gut and feed it what it needs. Whispers of intuition happen in the same way. If you are walking down an alley and you experience a feeling of danger, do you ignore it and keep walking? Perhaps in that moment you pause and assess the situation, you look around, you listen more closely, and you think harder about what direction you want to go next. You pause, and then, you take action! We need to take the same approach with feelings of inspiration or passion—let them speak to you, pause, and then take action.

; Not The End of Your Story

If you have come to a point of breakdown, a grey area, a loop in life, or simply a point where you feel you want something better for yourself—this is not the end of your story. This is just a chapter, a page, or a short sentence in it. You choose what gets written next. It's a story that has been told throughout time by different people, each telling complete with unique twists and turns. This is our opportunity to create the best version of life we can. Yes, we need to embrace change and advancement for all the good it brings to our world. But we cannot let those advancements come at the expense of other important things in our lives. We must continue using our minds, feeling with our hearts, and working with our hands. So let's roll up our sleeves, get our hands dirty, and dig into fixing the problems our lives have created.

If you feel drawn to act, you must ask the question—what are the actions you need to take? The answer will be different for everyone as we are all in a different place on this life journey. Some have traveled on the good path and will continue to do so. Look for those people and learn from them. Let their good words and actions guide you to the right path. We can all get lost at times and we need to look for the helpers, the dreamers, the leaders, and the visionaries. They are here to show us the way. They are here to share their words, music, art, and all the love in their hearts. They can lift us up and show us that there are better ways to live. You know these people; you know how you feel when you are around them and how they seem to brighten the room. Want to know a secret? That is what a good life looks like. It is not an exclusive club; it is not something out of your reach. You have that same potential within you. The goodness of what our life can be all comes down to the choices we make. If you've been on a path that led you to a broken reality, it's time to change directions. We can't change the past, but we can choose our next steps toward the future we want. Whatever path we've taken has been a choice, every single day and in every single way. Sure, there are experiences and moments we can't control, but our response is in our control! Yes, we are all broken but the power comes in healing what's broken and in piecing back the strong parts of ourselves in a new and beautiful way.

Our potential for success lives in our head and heart. We may have felt broken at times by the people, things, experiences, and circumstances of our story. Yes, we can all feel broken, but in healing what's broken and using the strong parts of ourselves—that's where power comes from. In my mind, life begins the day we heal and work through the brokenness from the past that is keeping us from being our best and most authentic selves. So, let's figure out how we can make better choices, how we can find our way and continue on a good path.

Your Next Step – Where Will Your Story Lead?

If you're feeling inspired but also a little lost, you are not alone. I was also lost when I started my journey of healing and self-discovery. The truth is, I am not here to give you all the answers to all the questions. Honestly, I don't have them. But I do hope my words lead you to feelings of motivation or discovery. To help you improve or make changes in your life, I've included a few instructions and tools to get you started on your journey of personal growth. What do you want to learn about or pursue next? What is the next helpful action to take to find a better version of life?

Consider this book a catalyst to discover your potential for happiness. Move forward with an open mind and heart, and the hope of good possibilities. So many people read self-help books, or listen to podcasts on personal growth, but how many take action to improve? I hope you'll choose to dig in and take action!

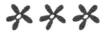

words to grow by

"The way I see it, if you want the rainbow, you gotta put up with the rain."

Dolly Parton

"Life is like a coin. You can spend it any way you wish, but you only spend it once."

Lillian Dickson

"Chaos in the world brings uneasiness, but it also allows the opportunity" for creativity and growth."

Tom Barrett

"Happiness is like a butterfly; the more you chase it, the more it will elude you, but if you turn your attention to other things, it will come and sit softly on your shoulder."

Henry David Thoreau

"The two most important days in your life are the day you are born and the day you find out why."

Mark Twain

Chapter 2
What Matters in Life

As we go through life, it's critical to identify and prioritize how we handle the things that matter. Have you ever stopped to think of what matters in your life? What are those essential pieces that are at the core of connecting us with ourselves and others? A lot of what matters in life is universal. If parts of your life are not working well, they may cause you to keep looping around and feeling stuck in life. These are the parts of life that I have come to realize matter most to me, and I'll share how I have worked to make these areas work better in life. These are they elements of life that make our days rich and worth living. Perhaps some of these will resonate with you as well.

Our Daily Routine Matters   Our Interpretation Matters
Our Thoughts Matter   Music & Media Matters
Our Mindset Matters   Community Matters
Our Words Matter   Relationships Matter

Our Daily Routine Matters

One day at a time—what can you do to make each day a good day? Having a daily routine or goal that focuses on our wellness is critical. One day at a time is all we should focus on. We can't go back to yesterday and we can't control tomorrow, so must learn to practice simply living for today. The journey to happiness doesn't happen all in one giant leap but rather in many small steps. As you figure out your next step, trust the process and know with each step it will improve your life and the lives of those around you. Over time you will realize that with each little step forward in the right direction, you will be making an impact on your life and experience for the good. So, choose how to spend your time wisely, and choose your actions with care.

Growth
Tool

Recipe For a Good Day

This won't be the recipe for everyone; think of it as a cheat sheet to consider, take ideas from, and adapt as needed. These are things (some little, some big) that have an impact on my wellbeing each day. To come up with your personal recipe, make a list of your daily habits. Consider the habits you've built that are not serving your wellness; the habits that are draining, stressful, or simply not providing you with good energy. Consider, too, any habits you used to have that you've stopped doing, particularly ones that helped you feel refreshed and focused. What opportunities are there for improvement? Perhaps it's something as simple as getting up when your alarm rings and not hitting snooze. Perhaps it's limiting time in front of the television and replacing it with reading. Write an outline or recipe for a good day and keep it somewhere where you look frequently to help remind yourself of your priorities. Once you identify the parts of your routine that are most important, you can more easily focus on them daily.

My Recipe for a Good Day
- Wake up
- Make my bed
- Get dressed

- Start my day with motivational or inspiring words or a happy song to set my energy or intention for the day
- Keep my work areas tidy and organized
- Achieve the work goals I set for that day by spending about the first 30 minutes triaging emails and my to do list and then prioritize what I need to do in that day
- Do something helpful for others
- Discover or learn something new such as an inspirational quote, a joke, a new song, a conversation with someone that challenges my thinking
- Be mindful of the money I spend compared to what I earn and save
- Interact with people outside my home
- At least 30 minutes of uninterrupted self-care
- Move my body
- Eat three healthy meals, and at least 1 meal around the table with the family
- Drink a healthy amount of water (discover your personal needs)
- One hour of unplugged time (no screens)
- Identify something from the day I was grateful for
- Good night of sleep (at least eight hours)

I also aim to be realistic, knowing there will be days when I don't fulfill every ingredient on my list. But I still strive to mark off as many as I can as often as I can. On the days or weeks when I struggle, I still reference my list to see the ingredients of a good day I've practiced and offer witness to the areas where I could improve.

Our Thoughts Matter

We have to be careful with our thoughts as they are the hinge to so many aspects in our lives. There is a quote by Lao Tzu you may have heard, but in case you haven't:

> *"Watch your thoughts, they become your words; watch your words, they become your actions; watch your actions, they become your habits; watch*

your habits, they become your character; watch your character, it becomes your destiny."

As humans, we can fall into harmful habits with our thoughts. When we allow ourselves to believe irrational and inaccurate thoughts, they can lead to so many problems in all aspects of our life. I call irrational thoughts the **Bullies in our Brains**. These bullies show up uninvited to punish and push us down, but only if we allow them.

Feed What You Want to Grow in Your Life

It takes five positive messages to erase one negative one. We have to be careful not to feed our mind's bullies. I believe in the power of positive thinking. Your mind will manifest what you feed it, whether it's self-critical thoughts, interpretation of the words and actions of others, the media you expose yourself to, or other outside sources. We have to choose what fills our life with care. Where your focus goes your energy flows. Feed your mind with all the good things in life:

- Hope
- Truth
- Love
- Kindness

With optimism comes strength, and in turn, even more success if we recognize challenges as opportunities instead of obstacles. We have more control of our lives than we realize, and the impact of our choices can change when we work from a healthier mindset. What choices will you make today and in the days ahead to improve your potential for better health, happiness, and stronger relationships? The first step may be to recognize what's in your mind, how it affects your view, and your response to it. Knowledge is power, so why not learn and grow?

There are two ways to look at this life and depending on your view, your experience is drastically affected. **Consider if you see your days as a time of growth and opportunity, OR do you focus on the limitations, obstacles, and things you can't control**. Did you know that perspective is in your control? Did you know you can work and strengthen your ability to see things differently? You can work to find more success, happiness, better health, and stronger relationships throughout your life. Are you feeding the positive thoughts, words, and actions or fueling the negative ones?

It's not too late to make changes whether big or small to make the days ahead better. Every interaction, word shared, or situation you experience is about you. Now, I'm not suggesting that you become a narcissist, rather, I'm hoping you realize the power and control you have over your life experience. It is about how you perceive it, how you respond to it, how you let it make you feel, how you let it control your thoughts, and how you take action each day. It is all about you, in the best ways, when you look at it from a perspective of growth and understanding. Don't undervalue yourself and how much control you have over everything that is coming your way right now. It all comes down to YOU! What will you choose? When you know better, you can do better. You control your mindset!

Our Mindset Matters

Whether you're an optimist or pessimist by nature, each of us has the opportunity to make good choices and find a healthy perspective and balance in life. It's the difference between a fixed mindset and a growth mindset. The difference between a positive attitude and a negative attitude. It's the difference in our choices each day.

Perhaps you've heard the story about the battle of two wolves that happens inside us all? There is a Cherokee legend about an elderly brave who tells his grandson about life. "Son," he says, "Within all of us there is a battle of two wolves. One is evil. He is anger, envy, jealousy, sorrow, regret, greed, arrogance, self-pity, guilt, resentment, inferiority, lies, false pride, superiority, and ego." He continued, "The other wolf is good. He is joy, peace, love, hope, serenity, humility, kindness, benevolence, empathy, generosity, truth, compassion, and faith." "The same fight is going on inside of you, and inside every other person, too," explained the wise Cherokee elder. The grandson thought about it for a minute and then asked his grandfather, "Which wolf will win?" The grandfather simply replied, "The one you feed."

In every choice and interaction, it is our choice what we feed. If we choose to feed the good, we can see improvement in our wellness and lives in general. If we choose good, we can work to enrich all areas of our wellness—physical, emotional, social, spiritual, intellectual, occupational, and financial. To find a healthy balance, we have to think it is possible to do so. We have to believe we are deserving and worthy of good feelings. What are things you do, or resources that help you find your balance and set your mind right?

Whether you've been told the number on the scale matters or not, imagine if instead of the weight of our body, a scale showed the weight of what was on our mind. Now that would be enlightening. The load we each carry is often more significant than we realize and may include:

- emotional problems
- personal responsibilities
- expectations from others
- stress of work
- negative or toxic media
- managing a household
- uncertainty
- life changes
- personal relationships
- financial security
- good health

Lighten what burdens you. Become aware of the things you should truly be carrying. No one is built to carry the world, let yourself set that load down. Now is a great time to pause and challenge our thinking, perceptions, and in turn our actions to reach the positive outcomes we'd like to see in our lives. We can't change how our story began. That's in the past. The good news is we absolutely can make an impact on today and the future! Life is what you manifest!

Life is all about choices, every day we each have many important ones to make. The wisdom comes in recognizing which are the most important ones and taking the right actions for the outcome you desire. A good place to begin practicing is when something bad happens. **In a bad situation, you have three choices: you can let it define you, destroy you, or you can let it strengthen you.** So much strength and growth can come from a positive mindset! Those two wolves are inside us all, and it is our choice to determine which wins. I hope you each navigate the choices in your daily life with care and can find your way to a path of wellness and all the good feelings!

Our Words Matter

In our society, we are often taught to show strength and knowledge in our communication and feel there is an expectation that it is best to be right. When faced with a situation where we don't know something, must admit we are wrong, or made a mistake it can feel like a moment of showing weakness. In these situations, many people get defensive and turn to unproductive communication. Too often, sharing words of emotional struggle or value are taboo. How often when someone starts to talk about feelings or sensitive experiences does it seem to make those in the room uncomfortable? Perhaps a sudden silence wraps the room when people don't know how to respond. Sometimes there is awkward laughter, a person who quickly tries to change the subject, or someone who immediately tries to put a positive spin on it. In those moments, if you are the one to speak up it can feel embarrassing, lonely, unsupported, and surely not a conversation you want to bring up again. Have we lost connection with sharing true words and feelings with one another for fear of being thought a fool or being judged? If we lose that connection, we lose humanity.

We need to be brave and communicate with strength and courage even if it reveals we need help or don't understand something. We need to be able to speak and listen with grace and compassion even if it reveals we are imperfect or at times we may be wrong. No one is right all the time. No one is perfect. No one is free of weakness. The sooner we remember that about ourselves the sooner we can listen to others with an open mind and kind heart. Truly listen and create a safe space for sharing. Instead of focusing on what we'll say, or how we'll respond, we need to hear each other first. Too often we think of how our words will help us get ahead, or how we can quickly defuse an uncomfortable situation. Through discomfort and choosing to continue the conversation we can better understand each other and grow as humans. How has the world become so narcissistic to think our perspectives or experiences are better or more important than those of our neighbors? That goes back to those thinking errors—the bullies in our brain. By speaking and sharing compassion with others it connects us.

Let's take another look at how we speak to others. Over time we often build negative habits in our communication. Again, going back to our pride and how we seem to focus so much on our personal perspectives. We all have perspectives but who is to say which is right and which is wrong. With most of life, there is not a clear right or wrong. Life isn't black and white; it is full of colors, and all have their beauty and value. The moment we stop seeing that rainbow of different views and perspectives we lose sight of each other.

The moment we can pause and try to see the viewpoint of others with an open mind and understanding heart the better conversations we can have. Consider this before you react to someone. **PAUSE. There is so much power in a pause.** A pause gives you a moment to think. A moment to consider what the other person may be thinking, feeling, or what has happened in their day or life leading up to this situation, leading up to this interaction or moment. Sounds like a super long and awkward pause, right? Unless you know everything about the person standing in front of you (or communicating through the screen)—their thoughts, feelings, and what's happened in their day or life in advance of that present moment—how could you possibly know their intention? Instead of an instant reaction, perhaps it's saying: "I need a moment to consider what you just said", "I need to gather my thoughts on that", "Give me a moment and I'll respond to your comment", "I'm not sure how to respond, can I clarify....?", or "that stirs up feelings and I need a moment to work through that before responding". Then take a big deep breath and consider what you'll say next. A pause does not mean you just stand and stare at them. That would be awkward.

Do you know what's great about realizing we don't know everything? We can pause instead to ask questions! Yes, those wonderful opportunities are there for us to ask instead of answer sometimes. To ask for clarification, to seek to understand better the words, actions, or interaction you are currently experiencing. Knowledge is power, and we can continue to seek it and grow! In every pause, you know what is the MOST IMPORTANT thing? Assume good intentions in others. Assume what they are saying is not meant to hurt you or push you down. Assume what they are saying, if not at first sounding kind, is coming from a place of hurt or misunderstanding in their life. So, in your response, respond to that underlying hurt, not to the words. I realize this is impossibly hard to imagine, but in simpler terms, as I know not everyone can sense the hurt and conflict in others—respond with kindness. Does any good come in creating conflict with our communication? Does any good come in arguing with negative words or putting down the thoughts of others? I'm not saying we'll always agree—we absolutely will not! We can disagree with respect. Often, we can agree to disagree and not simply disregard what the other person believes.

Sure, there are some very basic things we will all agree on—those have been the same basically since the beginning of time. The sky is blue. Grass is green. Treat people the way you want to be treated. Don't litter. The world is round. Those cannot be argued as some things there truly is only one right answer. We're not talking about those big things; we're talking about the little things here. Over time little interactions and misunderstandings become the big things. One small example of words that hurt our communication are the words *always* and *never*. Those words are likely ones we could remove from our language, and it would be a good improvement. Always and never are fitting examples of *overgeneralizations* and typically become fighting words as they put people on the defensive. Find ways to switch those words for more accurate quantifiers. With most things, always and never tends to be an exaggeration of the truth. The important thing is just as these bad communication habits were created; we can create positive communication with the same little steps. One thought, one word, one action, one day at a time.

Communicate with Good Intentions and Kindness, Not Judgment

Not sure what kind communication sounds like? It means we can disagree and still seek to understand the perspective of others. We can add to that perspective with our own and not have it be heard as a critique, judgment, or any inference of the other person being wrong. When we hear each other with good intentions and seek to understand another's perspective before responding with our own, it is easy to have a civil discussion that brings new information to the table for everyone.

Let me share a memorable example from the time I spent in the hospital. I was speaking with a gentleman who had schizophrenia. We had met and randomly got into a discussion about religion and politics, typically taboo subjects. This time it was the most amazing conversation and a couple of other gentlemen joined in. None of us agreed, but we all shared our unique perspectives. We listened to each other and opened our minds to hearing other points of view. There was no right or wrong, there was just a sharing of our thoughts and beliefs on the subjects. It was amazing and unexpected and really opened my eyes.

We went on to talk about the mental health stigma and how too often people with a diagnosis are labeled or judged based on that diagnosis. The man explained that his wife had cheated on him and left him because she couldn't handle his diagnosis. Sure, the guy had a rough past, but based on the stories he told and the fact he was seeking help it seemed to me he was working hard to turn his life around for good. It saddened me to hear how he seemed to be treated so poorly for things that were out of his control.

You see, some people have rough childhoods that don't set them up for an easy path to success. Some people struggle for years to get past their upbringing and learn new ways and better habits to find safety, good health, happiness, and success in their lives. I admire those people so much! In my mind, everyone's life begins the day they heal and work through all the baggage from the past that is keeping them from their potential and truer self.

I feel everyone is good at heart, but sometimes there are layers put around our heart to protect it, or hardship built into our genetics we must break down to reveal that goodness underneath. This man felt so much judgment and shame for his mistakes as a younger man before he found help. I shared my thoughts with him, and he seemed to appreciate the perspective like it was one he'd never heard or considered.

I hope everyone can work to judge less as we don't know the struggles of others. People have enough to carry without the added weight from the judgment of people in their lives. Our communication should show this compassion, grace, and understanding for others. Everyone has a story, and we are all at a unique chapter in ours. Will you lend kindness to the story of others as you cross paths, or will you add judgment?

Listen to the Words

I encourage you to listen for yourself as you read and to feel the words I share. Written words leave a lot to interpretation. The tone and intent behind the words can be missed. Over time this communication breakdown has led to misinterpretation which doesn't often end well. As you turn the pages, I hope you activate an awareness going forward to read with good intentions and feelings of kindness. This is my stone of kindness to throw in the ocean of hurt people are floating in and hope it makes a ripple of difference. I am just one little person, but I believe that's where it starts—

each of us realizing our power to make a difference in our little pond of influence. Please know that I am sending you strength to get over whatever molehill or mountain you face today. I am cheering for your success in life! If people can spread negativity and hate to strangers, I can send positive thoughts and love to those of you taking the time to read what I've written.

Our Interpretation Matters

So much of our lives are affected by our interpretation. Our personal evaluation dictates our response to everything we encounter and experience. Whether it's our actions, communication, relationships, career, mood, or attitude—they are all shaped and impacted by our interpretation of the world around us. Have you ever stopped to think about your interpretation of the exchanges, environments, and situations you encounter each day? How is it influencing your life? How does your perception impact your interpretation? What is the difference between perception and interpretation and how are they related? How do we gain control or change the way we interpret and experience things in our day-to-day life? Let's start by defining these terms.

Interpretation vs Perception
> per·cep·tion *noun*
> the ability to see, hear, or become aware of something through the senses.

> in·ter·pre·ta·tion *noun*
> the action of explaining the meaning of something.

The way I see it this is similar to the age-old question of which comes first, the chicken or the egg? Perception is about sensing and becoming aware of something. Interpretation is about explaining and deciphering meaning of the experience we are now aware of. Your interpretation can then bring a whole new set of feelings and thoughts. I think these two terms team up and work together, but I believe perception comes first. Once our senses are involved, they continue to play on the playground with the parts of our brain that are there to define and explain. The tricky thing about both is that they are very personal and can be quite subjective. Everyone has their own uniquely formed perception. Going back to the idea of the all-powerful pause, this is a great time to reengage that concept. When we perceive something, it engages our feelings, and our perception may trigger a strong reaction. At times that pause is our chance to assess if our feelings are valid or if there are other facts or details we need to assess before reacting based on our initial interpretation of the situation or conversation.

The Power of Thoughts and Feelings – A Checks and Balances System

What we think and feel is founded in our past experiences and should also be rooted in the evidence of our present, as well as the realistic hopes for our future. What we think and feel about ourselves comes to light in how we interpret and respond to the words and behaviors encountered with others. Any irrational thoughts or painful feelings introduced from experiences of someone's past hurt and misunderstandings can overthrow the current potential for understanding. Those strong feelings and memories can silence or conceal the facts of our current reality at times which leads to an inaccurate interpretation of the situation. If we work to heal from past hurt and build confidence in ourselves to take power back from the ugly self-doubt, judgment, fear, and irrational thoughts, we can change the narrative. By changing our narrative, we can interpret situations in a healthier way and respond in a more productive and balanced manner.

Remember those little bullies in our brain are constantly trying to take over. These bullies team up with our negative feelings to try to overtake us. This is where it is important to recognize that you have the power to bring balance back to your thoughts and feelings. If we don't balance ourselves with rational, constructive, and positive thoughts, those negative feelings start to win. I like to think of it as a checks and balances system. In one hand you have all your negative thoughts and feelings, in the other hand you hold your positive and productive thoughts and feelings. Each day we have to balance which side holds our strength and influence to respond in any given situation. When we let our negative feelings overpower our thoughts, we can feel unstable. If we let our unproductive thoughts overpower our positive feelings that can cause havoc as well. Our hearts and minds must work together. Both can be wrong at times so it's a sort of balance to check in with yourself and know where your reactions or responses are rooted. Are they rooted in truth or presumptions? Have they grown from facts or fictional interpretations? Identifying those bullies is important and allows us to set up a defense plan to keep them from winning.

In times of stress or conflict, the things that we've been bottling up can come flooding out. Feelings we've kept trapped inside or try to hide away may sneak out in ways we don't expect or even recognize. Our interpretation and response to the world around us needs to be balanced. You cannot see the truth in someone else's heart, so you cannot pass judgment on what choices in life are best for them. If their version of happiness doesn't inflict hurt on themselves or others, then who are we to judge? In this life, we all have choices to make and in the end our choices are up to us. Choose wisely.

The Impacts of Interpretation

When it comes to our language, we can speak and write with good intentions and still fall prey to misinterpretation. A saying that was on my parents wall when I was growing up that I will always remember explains it well.

"I know you may understand what you think I said, but what you do not realize is that what you heard is not what I meant."

At times misunderstandings can come from someone looking to pick apart a message; they might look for weakness or error in what was said and miss the meaning or value of the message because of one imperfect part. Other times words are heard through a filter of past hurt which can lead a person to assume the message is bad intentioned or cause them to respond aggressively or aversively. Why do people do this? Why do we ourselves do this at times? Well, it goes back to those words on how our thoughts matter. Our thoughts about past experiences affect our perspective, our perspective impacts our interpretation, which then influences our responses. Since we each have a unique perspective, if we're not careful with how we balance our past, present, and future realities we may choose to use our words and actions poorly. Poor choices in communication and behavior can lead to being misinterpreted or misinterpreting others.

Misinterpretation is substantially higher with written communication. Here we are reading the words of other people without being able to sense the full meaning behind the words they've used. We can't hear their tone, see their facial expression, recognize their eye contact, or notice their body language which are all telling components of language. It is much harder to interpret a person's emotions, attitude, or intention without these non-verbal attributes. We miss key factors of the message. In person, we are able to ask for clarification and more details if needed to fully decipher the message and better understand. We're all just winging it based on our unique perspectives and what we believe we interpret in the written words of others. This could be through email, text message, a handwritten note, or any other form of language shared where we miss the face-to-face benefits of communication. I believe that's part of why emojis have become helpful when used intentionally. They help impart the feeling behind the words typed. So, let's give each other room to improve, apologize, learn how to be better, and offer grace as we work to break some bad habits in our language and communication 😊.

Say What You Mean and Mean What You Say

Part of misunderstandings and misinterpretation is when we are not truthful or clear in how we communicate with others. Frustrations and hurt feelings come from moments and experiences where intentions and actions don't align. Sarcasm, inconsistencies, poor listening, not including all the necessary information, lying, or unclear explanations are all ways we can break down our chances of understanding one another. It goes back to the golden rule, treat others the way you want to be treated. Consider how you communicate with others as some day you may get a taste of your own medicine.

As with any medicine, language must be dispensed correctly. We've all heard the saying "a spoonful of sugar helps the medicine go down," but imagine the possibilities for misinterpretation without clarity in communication. If misunderstood, heaven knows where that spoon may go, and that could end in a much less positive experience if you ask me. Everyone could use a little more humor in life, so hopefully you heard the giggle behind that last line. We won't always get our words or message perfect the first time. Even Mary Poppins admits to only being practically perfect in every way, so why should we expect anyone to be perfectly perfect. Offer grace, ask for clarification, seek to understand—then respond. That's what the pause is for.

Do you know the saying you attract more bees with honey? For so long I've been saying to make it a sweet life. With sweet words and actions, we can enjoy a sweeter time together. I understand these words may seem like they are dripping in sugar, but I'm not sugarcoating it. This is the honest to goodness truth of how sweet and good life could be if people would— PAUSE—and consider how they are communicating with each other. It doesn't matter what language you're speaking; we all speak the human language. A language that in any translation can speak of kindness, compassion, and understanding. With all the advancements we're making, let's use our editing skills a bit better. Can you find that delete button? No? What about the backspace? Ah yes, there it is. That, my friends, is the key to change. **To change our language, we need to delete the negativity and back up from the judgment.** I'm not saying to erase everything written or spoken in our past. Not at all. I'm asking us to learn from it. There's space for a lot of things in life, and learning from past misunderstandings, mistakes, and misinterpretations is part of our big story. All good stories start somewhere, and I hope you'll choose to keep reading and find where this new path leads you. Even if you have chosen a path of negativity and judgment in the past, today is a new day and an opportunity to move forward on a path of healing, positivity, growth, and understanding.

Music & Media Matters

Many great things have been shared in books, songs, poems, and so many more ways. Throughout time music and media have had more power in our lives than we often credit. The visionaries, dreamers, innovators, and storytellers of the past had amazing works that came from a variety of experiences that shaped where we are today. Some say music can speak to the soul and be felt more deeply than any spoken word. Music can communicate to and for our hearts when we can't find the words. If music has such power, have you considered if we are using its power for good?

Music, books, and art are all threads in the tapestry of our history. Each tells a story of our past and often they reflect the thoughts and feelings of those times. The reality is not all of our past was good, and that is reflected in what came out of those times. We should not hide those away or pretend they didn't happen, but instead, learn from them and grow. We can read, listen, and look at the works that came from various times in history with an open mind and pull out the pieces that could be helpful in our life. Let music, media, and art speak to your heart. If you feel sad or lonely, listen to music that will lift your spirits. Pick up a book and be transported to a different time or place through the carefully crafted written imagery. Visit an art gallery and go on a visual journey through the strokes of a paintbrush or the moments captured in a photo. Know what chapter of your life you are in and play, read, or look for what your heart needs.

Of all the creative works, music is one of the most healing for me. It is interesting how I can listen to the same song at different times in my life, and it will be a unique and different experience in what I feel as I listen. Music can hold memories. Certain songs can bring you back to a time or place when you hear them. If you're married, you may have a wedding song. I know my parents' wedding song. I have memories of it from childhood; whenever it came on, they would dance or share a kiss. So, if I hear "Can't Help Falling in Love," sung by Elvis Presley, I pause and think of the love shared between my parents. Right now, it makes me feel a bit sad to hear this song since the last and most recent memory I have of my parents' hearing it was when my dad was dying of brain cancer. In time, I know the sadness of that memory will transition and again be overwhelmed by the happier memories of the past. Until then, I can allow myself to feel that grief and sadness; I hold space for it and allow it to sit with me.

Music can also inspire reflection or acknowledgment of feelings we didn't realize we'd buried. I often lean into music to allow me to connect with my feelings or to help push me out of a funk. One song that strikes a chord is "She Used to Be Mine" by Sara Bareilles. These lines of lyrics especially:

> *"She's imperfect but she tries*
> *She is good but she lies*
> *She is hard on herself*
> *She is broken and won't ask for help*
> *She is messy but she's kind*
> *She is lonely most of the time*
> *She is all of this mixed up*
> *And baked in a beautiful pie*
> *She is gone but she used to be mine"*

I heard this song at a time when I was struggling and felt like I had lost myself. She touches on the feelings of feeling lost in the shuffle of life and feeling unseen, unappreciated, broken, and alone. The lyrics connected with me at a core level in the years I had neglected self-care for so long. I took care of everyone and everything else in my life, so much so that I didn't recognize myself. I was going through the motions and felt like I had lost the passion and fire inside me.

When there are times that my flicker of passion is struggling, it may sound silly, but a good singing or dance break does wonders for my mood. Some of my favorites to help me feel strong and empowered to take that next breath; songs like "Respect" by Aretha Franklin, "Stronger" by Kelly Clarkson, "Roar" by Katy Perry, "F'ing Perfect" by Pink, "I Will Survive" by Gloria Gaynor, "Broken & Beautiful" by Kelly Clarkson, "Brave" by Sara Bareilles, "Better When I'm Dancing" by Meghan Trainor, and last but not least, "SexyBack" by Justin Timberlake. If you don't already have one, create your own power song playlist. When you feel yourself looping or sinking into a negative spiral, take a few deep breaths, pull out that song list, and play it loud. Dance it out if the mood strikes you.

Negative Media in Our Life

Don't allow society to hinder your dreams, nor the media to obscure your vision. It is important that we pay more attention to what we're choosing to listen to, watch, and share. An example, I quit watching the nightly news years ago as I found much of what was shared to be unhelpful. So much of the focus is on the bad. Why not share more of the good? This world is full of SO MUCH good! Why are we not sharing and celebrating it more? We tell our children we are here to protect them, to protect their minds and eyes from things that could hurt them. Why do we hold ourselves in less value? Do we think as we've matured somehow our minds work differently? We have pushed ourselves down with negativity for too long, and it has affected our society in ways we didn't realize. It is time to wake up and make a change. Where our focus goes our energy flows, so we need to be mindful of what we are focusing our time on.

Many of the words and images we view and share through the news, on television, and on our screens in general are hurting us. It is changing our relationships and our perspective on the world. Looking back in history, there were times where more wholesome content and messages were being shared to "entertain us." Perhaps the storytellers of our past weren't creating for entertainment, but to educate and teach us a way of life. Life doesn't come with an instruction manual. We are born and it's on-the-job training from there. Sink or swim—it's up to us. Let's work harder to enrich and entertain our lives in healthier ways.

Let's bring back news stories that show helpers doing good in their communities. Let's have television programs that offer images of how to be a good friend, a good neighbor, a good parent, a good spouse, and a good human. Let's have songs that encourage love and kindness. Songs to empower our days and actions. Songs that remind us how easy it can be to communicate, connect, and love others. Let's tell stories of great adventures, friendships, and life. As artists continue to share the beauty of the world through their eyes, may they see the good and enrich it with all the beautiful colors this world has to offer. We need all these perspectives to fill our hearts and minds with the potential and the truth of what we can be.

Community Matters

Communities Are as Strong as Its Members

In other times, people held greater regard for the value of connecting with their neighbors and asking for help when they needed it. If a crop was ready and would go to waste unless harvested, the community would rally together to help. Not because they were getting paid, not because they were getting grand recognition for helping, but because it was the neighborly and good thing to do. In modern times, life is busier. We have more things to juggle, but we must remember that we are one small piece of the puzzle. If we aren't doing our part to contribute to the whole, it is incomplete. Sure, there may not be as many family farms or crops to harvest, but there are worthy causes in every community where people can work together. Sharing and showing up for others with support matters! People from all walks of life, strangers even, can come together to show care and help one another.

It doesn't have to be grand; it can be the simplest action. Let's start right next door. Do you know your neighbor by their first name? Do you have their phone number so you can text them or call if you need a cup of sugar? If not, why wait to make that connection? For goodness sakes, if we can't reach out to those who live right next door, who can we reach out to? I'm not saying you must be besties who hang out every Friday, but let's be honest, it might be a little amazing if that were the case, right? Okay, maybe it's just me; I'm a bit of an extrovert, so the thought of a weekly happy hour makes me do a little happy dance. I get it though, we're all different, and for you, that may sound less than fun. It's cool, but that shouldn't stop you from reaching out to those in your community.

Community gives us connection. It gives us a way to relate with something bigger than ourselves. In connecting with others, we can more fully live our best life. We can share our gifts with others, we can share in the human experience, we can help each other to walk through this journey of life. When we can, we help! Consider the gifts you can offer in your community. If you have an abundance of something, why not share it? Now don't read this as meaning you have to give away all your money and possessions. A gift could be your time, talent, a listening ear, or a thoughtful offer to help a neighbor. Everyone can lend a little sweetness to the life of those around them. A hand outreached with care makes all the difference. People like to feel useful, helpful, and needed; we like to feel seen, that we belong, and are a part of something.

So next time you go to the mailbox or see each other as you head out your doors—pause for a moment and engage. Each kind word or action you toss out into your small community matters. The world is full of different little communities that together can make a big happy family when we support each other in both good and challenging times. We know this is true, otherwise, why would we keep telling stories and sharing phrases about pebbles being thrown in ponds to make a ripple? Or starfish being thrown back into the ocean? Or all those fish in the sea? You see, that's what we're here for. It's about something bigger than us, and that ripple of love can start with one kind touch, thought, word, or action. Positivity and kindness are more powerful than we realize! Over time, strong communities can begin to feel like family—a family you choose to have in your life.

Push past the fear of what others will think. If you are sharing words or actions with good intentions, what can it hurt? Perhaps you didn't grow up in a family or neighborhood that was very involved in the community you lived in. It may feel odd. But sharing your presence is not odd; it allows the most amazing feeling! Your life is meant to be shared with those around you! If this is new to you, it may be hard to take the first step. It may feel uncomfortable. Don't back down from the awkward and uncomfortable. Out of awkward moments can come the most beautiful relationships. Think back to your first kiss or first date. It likely wasn't your most magical and confident moment, but would you have just walked away instead of trying? Not every interaction can be a success. Sometimes we swing and miss, but we must keep swinging. Not sure where to start? Keep reading for ideas to get your inspiration flowing.

The Value of Community

We all have neighbors in life. I think of a neighbor as more than someone who lives next door. Neighbors are the people that are part of our larger community. I also consider neighbors to be the people we associate with online. The world as we experience it can be small, and what began as an online connection could end up becoming a next-door neighbor, or someone you might work with in the future. Every human we interact with deserves kindness. Here are some quick examples from my life. After my car accident, a mailwoman I had never met but had connected with through a couple of online groups brought me a beautiful flower arrangement. A new neighbor I'd met at a caroling event I hosted brought me a mug and sweet treats. Another neighbor, whose husband coached my son's soccer team a few years back, saw me at the library and offered me a hug and a few compassionate words. To be honest, I don't think all of them knew I had been in an accident. One did. And perhaps the mailwoman noticed I wasn't checking my mailbox for a while as mail piled up. And the new neighbor likely noticed I had been quiet on social media for a while as I am an almost daily poster. Yet I'd met each of these people in different ways and had different levels of connection. I consider them all to be people in my "neighborhood" who each offered caring and thoughtful actions.

Growth
Tool

Ways to Share and Build Community

Consider what makes a good neighborhood. What can each of us do to nurture the kind of community we want in our lives?
- If you are on a walk and see another person, smile. Say hello.

- Perhaps you love to garden and have a bouquet of flowers you could deliver to a neighbor to brighten their day.

- If you are heading into town and know an elderly neighbor has trouble running errands, why not ask if you can pick something up for them while you're out?

- If you are going to the park with your kids and know a neighbor is busy working on a project, offer them a break and ask if their kids can join you.

- If a new person or family moves into the neighborhood (or joins an online community), why not bring a goodie basket or offer a kind note welcoming them to the community?

- If you are interested in something, share it, and invite others to join you (potluck at the park, evening stroll through neighborhoods, quick pick-up game of kickball with friends).

Looking for ways to build community? Here are some ideas to get your inspiration flowing: walking group, cat lovers' coffee chat, gardening group, book club, knitting group, hiking group, happy hour club, Sunday scavenger hunt (a group of families and it can rotate who organizes the scavenger hunt), soup Saturday (a group of friends meets at one person's house, which rotates each week for a simple night of soup and conversation). Your options are limited only by your imagination.

If there isn't a group that fits your style of community, create one! People are inclined to seek out others with similar interests. So, look for what you want or create what you want. This is one of the ways I like to use social media. Yes, social media isn't for some people, but I have found it to be amazing for connecting with people and groups in my community. As with the other parts of life, you get back what you put in; when you choose to engage in good and helpful ways online, it can help contribute to positive personal growth and connections.

Of course, there might be times when budgets are tight, or time may be short. We should feel comfortable looking to our community for support. We should not be too proud to mention when we are struggling and seek help. We all need help sometimes. Why struggle when there are good people that want to see you succeed. Push your pride aside if it's getting in your way and see the potential to have honest connections with those around you.

It takes a powerful ship to get through a storm at sea. We should not feel like we're in our own little lifeboat. We need to support each other to get through each passing wave and help each other hold on to hope. There's no use breaking away and doing it all alone. Find or build your community group, your own close circle of people. Find your ship. No one should be rowing through this storm alone. Reach out or up! Don't stop reaching!

A community can look different for different people too, whether it be in person or online. This is the wonderful thing about advancement and change; with modern technology, there are countless ways to stay connected with the people, places, and things we care about. For me, in person is best. I don't often turn down an opportunity for face-to-face as opposed to a screen in my face. For others, especially after a pandemic experience, there can be hesitation to be back in person. Anxiety about being with groups of people face-to-face. In those situations, I am so thankful for the option of connecting through a screen. Without community, it can be isolating and lonely, and no one should be left out of the good feelings that come from connection.

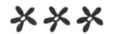

Chapter 3
All About Relationships

Life brings us many relationships, and one of the best things we can do to enrich our experience is to develop and strengthen the relationships that matter. As we age, our responsibilities increase, free time decreases, and the measure of relationships changes. Life is personal, it is not a business, but we should absolutely look at the "Return on Investment" of our relationships and evaluate whether we have good partners in life. Equitable relationships with mutual understanding and common values are priceless and worth taking stock in. Relationships come into our lives for a reason, a season, and sometimes a lifetime. Each holds exceptional value, and like most things, it is about quality, not quantity!

Happy Spouse Happy House

Our relationships are weighed against all the activities and distractions that we fill our lives with. At times we can get so busy that we forget to prioritize and be available for what matters. If we're honest, those distractions and activities are often just our excuses. There is no excuse for not making your relationship a priority! Whether the relationship is a man and a woman, a woman and a woman, a man and a man, or a family that has been broken and becomes complete by combining households in one larger loving family. However the love story is told in your home, you can choose to prioritize where, with whom, and how you spend your time and energy. Think back to what I've already shared on thoughts, words, and language, and then read on with an open mind and heart.

Have you ever considered the ways our world has advanced and evolved, yet somehow the expectations in our relationships have not transformed alongside those changes? We must reconsider the ways in which we structure our households. Spouses often both work and share the load of each managing a job and a family. As such, the management and workload of the home must be shared as well. What a happy family looks like will be different in each home. It's time to move past the old standard gender roles and develop new ones that will work to strengthen our homes and families. To do so, we need to revisit some of the basics of effective communication and consider ways in which we can support one another as these are two of the biggest foundations of a healthy and happy relationship.

Communicate with Empathy, Compassion, and Openness

As we dig into communication within our relationships it is helpful to define some of these words as we will use them often:

em·pa·thy *noun*
the ability and desire to understand and share the feelings of another, to see yourself in someone else's shoes

com·pas·sion *noun*
concern for the experience or situation of others and a desire to help

o·pen·ness *noun*
acceptance of or receptiveness to change or new ideas, lack of secrecy

In a romantic partnership, it is imperative to open yourself to the act of vulnerability. Too often our communication, or lack thereof, leaves too much room for misunderstandings. These misunderstandings often come from a breakdown in open, honest, kind, supportive, and understanding communication. Often time, an inability to share yourself fully comes from feelings of anxiety around judgment, fear, or shame. It is the big communication breakdown in our lives that is breaking our families. Relationships in the home are at the heart of our lives.

How do we start to heal broken communication habits? First, be courageous and speak up, with kindness, when things feel amiss. Don't wait until the dust settles to pull up that rug. Shake the rug out every day! Shake it out when you notice a crumb. Don't let the crumbs settle—they will become embedded into the fabric. Unspoken, our thoughts will manifest in ways that do not serve our relationships. Our partner cannot read our thoughts, anticipate our needs, or understand every value we hold in our hearts unless we communicate them. We need to take it upon ourselves to speak up and share ourselves. We need to advocate for what we need. Don't hide your pain, and don't shy away from sharing your successes out of fear of how your partner will respond. Did you pause to consider they may be feeling vulnerable too?

And it must go both ways. If you stop and ask questions and work to understand what is truly in your partner's heart and mind, you will better hear them. If you share more of what you are feeling without the worry of pride or perfection, they can better understand you too. If either person is focused only on being heard or being "right," half the message is lost, and we all know a one-sided conversation isn't much help. There are two sides to every conversation. We must take the time to listen, truly listen, and make attempts to understand before we speak. If we don't understand, we must be courageous enough to ask for clarification and keep asking until we understand more clearly. Before we speak, we must consider how our words may be received. In fact, slight changes to our communication may allow *our* message to be heard more clearly. In turn, we'll both find greater understanding and potential for growth.

One thing I learned when I was trained as a Peer Conflict Mediator that has helped my communication skills was the value of **"I statements"** instead of **"you statements,"** which is a style of communication first explored by

Thomas Gordon.*[1] It made such a difference in how I approached emotional conversations and alleviated some of the risks of the other person responding defensively. "I statements" allow you to be assertive with your communication without making accusations. It's ultimately a matter of identifying and acknowledging our own feelings rather than leading with any assumptions, judgments, beliefs, or valuations we may have made about the other person's thoughts, feelings, or experience. It's best not to assume your partner intended for their actions to cause bad feelings, and this method of communication allows you to converse in a way that lets your partner know how you feel and how their behavior has affected you.

As I mentioned in the Our Words Matter section of this book, avoid using "always" or "never" or other statements that generalize. Below are tips to start healing broken communication habits.

Growth Tool

How to Use I Statements

If you are not familiar with "I statements," here are a few examples. Let's practice together. The trick to make this work:

> **I feel** <insert your actual feelings>
> *Avoid using I-statements to express anger. Instead, learn to express the deeper feelings (hurt, frustration, fear, disappointment) before you get angry.*
> **when** <insert their action or behavior that led to your feeling>.

Here are some examples:

1. Try saying, "I feel frustrated when you say you'll do the dishes and don't follow through," instead of, "You make me so mad because you never do the dishes when you say you will."

2. Try saying, "I feel disconnected and lonely when you don't respond to my messages," instead of, "You always ignore me."

---

[1] Resources included at end of book

3. Try saying, "I feel disrespected and hurt when you raise your voice at me and it makes me not want to continue talking," instead of, "You make it so I can't even talk to you."

Write Your Own _____

_____

Want to take it a step further? Add a potential solution:
> **I feel** <insert your actual feelings>
> **when** <insert their action or behavior that led to your feeling>
> **next time** <insert what you need or want and how that would make you feel in a positive way>.

Here are some examples:

1. "I feel frustrated when you say you'll do the dishes and then don't follow through. Next time when you say you'll help, it would make me feel supported if you did it."

2. "I feel disconnected and unimportant when you don't respond to my messages. In the future, I would feel more valued and cared for if you responded to my messages."

3. "I feel disrespected and hurt when you raise your voice at me. I need you to lower your voice so I feel more comfortable speaking with you."

Write Your Own _____

_____

For those that read these examples and find a way around the examples—I will also point out what _not_ to do.

An "I statement" is NOT:
> "I feel like you are being a jerk."
> "I feel like you never listen."
> "I think you are being irresponsible."

Can you see what is missing in each of these statements? Although each statement begins with "I feel" and "I think," none of them include feeling statements. These examples do not allow vulnerability to be part of the conversation. Focus on the way an action affected you and how it made you feel.

Growth Tool

Why to Avoid Why Statements

Another great tool to foster productive communication involves **avoiding "why statements."** When you phrase something as a "why statement," it assumes the other person is guilty, which is likely to put them on the defensive and may bring about a combative reaction. This is another opportunity to use an "I statement" instead.

Here are some examples:

1. Instead of, "Why are you always on your phone?" try saying, "I feel lonely when you are focused on your phone when we are together."

2. Instead of, "Why don't you find me attractive?" try saying, "I feel unwanted and undesired when you don't initiate physical intimacy with me."

3. Instead of, "Why don't you like anything I do?" try saying, "I feel embarrassed and sad when you criticize me."

Write Your Own _____

_____

Now take it a step further—offer a solution:

1. "I feel lonely when you are more focused on your phone than me when we are together. In the future, I would feel happier if we could set some boundaries on phone usage so we can enjoy more quality time together."

2. "I feel disconnected and undesired when you don't initiate physical intimacy with me. In the future, it would help me feel seen and desired if you reached to hold my hand, gave me a kiss, or a hug."

3. "I feel embarrassed and sad when you criticize me. I would feel more appreciated if you could say more positive things about me."

Write Your Own _____

_____

Growth Tool

Learning To Speak with Love

Although I knew how to use "I statements" from an early age, I have not always used them regularly in my own relationships. There are wonderful ways to use variations of "I statements" to advocate for what you need when there is a not a conflict as well.

Reminder: humans can't read minds. Here are some ideas of positive ways we can ask for what we need using examples of the **5 Love Languages.**[*2]

Physical touch: "I am feeling sad and would love a hug."

Acts of service: "I am feeling overwhelmed and would really appreciate it if you could help fold laundry."

Quality time: "I am feeling anxious; could we put down our phones and go for a walk?"

Words of affirmation: "I am feeling discouraged, can you remind me what you love about me?"

Receiving gifts: "I feel so loved when you surprise me with flowers."

Write Your Own _____

_____

Although these examples assume a partnership, "I statements" can be helpful in communicating with our children and other loved ones. It can be easy to fall into ineffective communication habits and defensive mechanisms that build over time. If I had been more confident in the early years of my marriage to speak up and confront conflict, I could've avoided a lot of loneliness, pain, and resentment. If I had worked harder to have productive conversations with my partner, I would've felt more heard and understood. The foundations of communication between my husband and I

---

[2] Resources included at end of book

were challenging in part due to my avoidance of conflict and my inability to talk through my feelings. I made the mistake of assuming instead of asking. Often my husband would say something, and I would take offense, thinking he was criticizing me. I would shut down and become defensive. Instead of pausing to ask for clarification, or pausing to remember he had good intentions, I broke down. If he spoke passionately about something, or we disagreed, often I would cry. When I cried or shut down, he would get upset as it put a stalemate to whatever conversation he was trying to have.

Growing up I can't remember a time when I saw my parents argue or fight. So, when my husband and I experienced disagreements, I assumed it was a failure in our marriage and a failure of me as a wife. In those early years, my communication skills lacked openness and emotional awareness, a fact that is easy for me to see today. I had a case of you don't know until you know. I now realize that disagreements can lead to relationship growth when they're explored with respect, empathy, compassion, and kindness. It is not necessarily a sign of failure. Growth requires change, which can be hard. The important thing to remember is almost every issue or conflict in a relationship is caused by both people to some degree. To move forward takes the effort, commitment, and love of both people.

Acknowledging your feelings and the action(s) that led to them will make it easier to work toward a solution. This process can allow us to talk more openly and look for compromises, or at least learn more about our partner and how our interactions impact each other. Today is an excellent day to start talking about the things that matter. And it's okay if you need to reach out for help. You are not alone— I'm still learning too! Relationship coaches or therapists are an amazing resource to help you dive into what may be holding you back. They can help you break down those walls of communication.

Is The Mental Load Weighing You Down?

Life comes in waves and at times it can feel as though we are being asked to do more than we can. And the biggest weight is often the mental load. Have you heard of this term? If not, the simplest way I can explain it is **the mental gymnastics we go through trying to anticipate everyone else's needs, making plans to meet those needs, and assigning tasks to ensure it all gets done.** The mental load can be exhausting if not shared. If you share a home or life with someone and haven't already, it's important to talk about this load with those you live with so you can work together to help carry that weight. The mental load is something that happens in life whether you expect it or not. It happens in everyday life, and it is women who often take on the brunt of its burden.

I was recently talking with a friend about how we all have a mental load that we're carrying around. We talked about how it can be hard to let go of tasks out of fear. Fear it won't get done in the time frame or way we prefer. Fear it will be done incorrectly or won't get done and we'll end up having to do it anyway. Or fear that someone else can do it better than us and we'll feel inadequate. There is always fear, but fear is what holds us back from opportunity. If your mental load is not sustainable; you must let go of your fears and lessen your load. Replace fear with trust and a heap of realistic expectations (I'm talking to the perfectionists here, especially). Here's a great quote by Lena Horne, "It's not the load that breaks you down, it's the way you carry it." Acknowledging when that load is putting a strain in areas that could be relieved if carried differently offers an opportunity to work on shifting your form, changing your habits, or simply shaking things up.

With a household mental load, you must accept that some tasks will be done differently by other members in the household. The towels may be folded differently. The grass may be mowed shorter than you prefer. The dishwasher may be loaded in a new way, or family recreation may be planned in ways you didn't expect. You may have to take deep breaths trusting your partner can manage sports schedules even if you don't get the team communication. Groceries may get put away in various places, and the bills may get paid on a different day. Trust that these differences are okay and may be necessary. To share the load, you must be willing to let go a little, or sometimes a lot.

This is just the tip of the iceberg on what some of you may be carrying. Don't wait for an avalanche before talking to your spouse. There is no prize or first place ribbon for you if you choose to take on all the tasks of maintaining your home alone. It's not sustainable and can lead to resentment over time. Your family may not even realize what you're carrying. If you do a "good job," it may seem effortless to others. Another thing to consider—your spouse is carrying their own mental load. Again, unless you talk about these things, that lack of understanding and support from each other adds unnecessary stress to a relationship.

Growth Tool

Continue - Drop – Swap Exercise

Not sure where to start? Start by making a list of the things you manage for your household and ask your partner to make a list too. Have a conversation about what each of you is doing. What are you comfortable continuing to do? Discuss and decide together if certain things should be dropped from either of your lists. Does every task provide enough value to your family? If one of you is feeling overwhelmed or buried by your list, talk about what may need to be swapped off to the other partner. If you are the one swapping something, ask if they want to hear how you've done it before, or if they prefer to come up with their own processes. Now you have a new framework—**continue, drop, swap**—and then move forward.

When learning to do new things, at some point, we all fail. Offer each other grace and loving encouragement as you work to share the load. If it gets done and you can take it off your task/stress list—that is the goal! Don't let the method make you mad, focus on the goal being accomplished and be glad for the help. If you critique or nitpick each other that adds new weight to that emotional load. So don't get caught doing that! Once you improve your communication and support of each other in even these two small ways, it may open some more good feelings between you. If done right, it can crack away at feelings of resentment and loneliness. Remember, it's not a one-and-done process. Keep checking in. Keep shaking out that rug. Let's love and be loved in the best ways we know how. We deserve all the good feelings!

Feeling Good Like We Should

Speaking of staying in touch and feeling all the good feelings, let's not forget the importance of intimacy. At the beginning of a romantic partnership, things are often hot and steamy. Perhaps you're the couple that couldn't keep your hands off each other. As relationships mature, that initial hot burn can simmer, but there should always be something sizzling under the surface. Maybe you don't hold hands as much, or perhaps that kiss goodnight has been forgotten. Closeness and physical touch can be a way to connect, and sometimes, especially those with young kids, that closeness gets further and further away. After having kids poke and pull at you all day it can reach a point of sensory overload. Some call this being "touched out" or sensory exhaustion. At times, by the end of the day, once back together with a partner, advances may get rejected for this reason. If feelings of rejection aren't talked about, it can result in a blow to self-confidence and discourage future advances.

If you feel disconnected, start small. Yes, talk, and begin to take steps to reconnect. Choose to sit next to your partner on the couch. Reach to hold their hand, put a hand on their leg or over their shoulder. Initiate a kiss and make it better than the kiss you'd give your grandma for goodness sake. An intimate kiss should last a few seconds, even a few seconds of physical contact can initiate a level of closeness a simple peck won't. It doesn't necessarily need to lead to more, but it may help reignite that sizzle. Next time you go in for a hug, embrace a bit longer, and hold them a bit tighter. Also, sometimes we need to ignore our pride; it can be easy to assume the other person should initiate. Let's not make it a game of chicken and stall out with neither of you taking the opportunity to move toward each other. No one wins then.

Start small. Those slight changes will help you build a stronger connection. Adults should be reaping more benefits from communicating and working to understand the needs of one another in the bedroom. We deserve to experience and feel all the good things in life. What worked at one point may not work later, and when life gets busy, you may have to talk about how you can make intimacy a priority. I know it doesn't sound romantic or sexy, but there's nothing sexy about being disconnected from your partner either. Don't be afraid a conversation will make it awkward in the bedroom. Talk about your feelings, fears, and what you want and need. Talk about what feels good and what doesn't—talk about it all!

As a woman and mother of three, I know that body insecurity can be an unwelcome guest in the bedroom. Motherhood or not, our bodies change with time. It can be hard to see ourselves as beautiful with the new sidekick of stretch marks, saggy skin, wrinkles, or whatever other changes we feel self-conscious about. It can feel embarrassing or unattractive to think of being stripped bare in front of our partner. If you have similar thoughts or feelings, this is a case of those bullies in our brain picking on us. If you are with someone you love and who loves you, believe me, they are not looking at you naked and judging you. They are wanting to love every inch of your body. Maybe I'm getting too personal, but goodness, if you can't be personal with the person you are connecting with in the bedroom (or whatever room in the house you prefer), you might have to reconsider your priorities.

I know sex has been called many names in our history to try to lighten the mood. Let's not forget what it's all about shall we? It's making love folks, plain and simple. For a family to grow, it helps to start from a place of love. If you're not in love, you shouldn't be doing it. If you are deeply in love, you should do it as often as you want. And in a loving relationship, we must learn not to take it personally if and when our partner is not in the mood. You can respond from a place of compassion and understanding, knowing if the situation were reversed, you will receive the same loving response in return.

Enough of all that making whoopie business, and honestly, can we agree that "sex" doesn't sound pleasant to say? It doesn't roll off the tongue with ease if you ask me. Okay, okay, getting a little too hot and steamy now. This isn't that kind of a book. That said, there is a lot to talk about regarding sex. There are many experts out there— look for resources and don't be too shy to reach out for help. As I mentioned before, everyone can share their passion and expand their knowledge. A helpful resource to learn about how to better communicate in the bedroom comes from Vanessa and Xander Marin,*[3] two wonderful sex therapists who provide raw and real resources.

One last thing, what happens in the bedroom (or whatever other room in the house) should stay there. That is a special loving act between two people and some things aren't meant to be shared. Sharing is only caring if you do it with love and good intentions.

The Family Connection

The special bond in a family is just that, special. Don't let others break that bond. Don't let anyone or anything interfere with that connection you have.

---

[3] Resources included at end of book

If we let distractions get in the way of our bonds, they can break down over time. Sure, with some tools you may be able to repair that bond if your foundation is strong and can hold the extra weight. But is that a chance you want to take? Why are we sitting beside someone we care about with our eyes on our screens instead of looking into the eyes of our family members? Why are we sitting in the same room with each other and busy having conversations with people outside of our household? Why are we letting our feelings and actions stray away from the ones we should be showing the most love to? These actions can hurt the quality of our relationships and the health and happiness of our families.

The duties and responsibilities of life should not have priority over the people in our home. Let's bring love, respect, and attention back where it matters. Let's quit breaking the foundation of what keeps this world strong. Everything has its core, its heart, and our families are at the heart of everything. Every family, whether blended or not, has its core. The adults in the house who are setting the boundaries and communicating the expectations for the home set the tone. You should show up to bat every day and focus on the work of fostering the health and happiness of your home. There's no magic trick or big secret to make this happen, it takes work. It is worth every effort, and it is important.

Life is busy, and there are times when you will need to divide and conquer to meet everyone's needs. But when you're together, as a family, find ways to be together in all the ways. Sit at the table together to eat a meal. It might not always happen around the table, so let's not be too rigid with our ideals. Some of my favorite memories growing up occurred on the road with my family. My parents would pack plenty of food. When our stock ran short, my dad would stop for ice cream sandwiches when we would stop to refuel. We would often have a family movie night on the weekends and sometimes we'd go a little crazy and eat nachos or pizza by the TV together. That was a special thing I looked forward to. Other favorite activities involved packing up to have a picnic in a park or loading up our gear and heading to the beach. Make time for special moments and special meals together.

A family meal—sometimes it's simple and sometimes it's not. Meals are usually not picture-perfect. You may hear complaints about the meal, and most times reminders on manners are needed. That is also part of family life and how kids learn how to be good humans and respectful guests in others' homes. Don't give up on family meals and remember we are teaching children by example. We are showing them what a happy and healthy family looks like and acts like. We are showing them with our example and actions what the priorities in life are. Meals are just the beginning, there are many other things to teach when they are young. When we get right down to it, most of us only get about 18 years with our kids living under our roof. That time goes fast. We need to make the most of our time. We aren't simply raising children; we are raising future adults.

Raising Future Adults

If you got to this section and don't have kids, you may think this is one to skip. Please don't. Whether you have kids or not, we are all responsible for helping to teach the next generation, to raise these future adults. Whether it be the neighbor kid, a niece or nephew, a grandchild, or your friend's little one—you are a part of their life. You have an influence, so make sure it's good. Back in the day, the saying "it takes a village to raise a child" was the norm. Why have we moved away from that? Yes, I realize there are a variety of parenting styles but aren't there basics we can agree on? Shouldn't we model and encourage the things that matter in our interactions?

Let's do the work to protect children from what may hurt them but not shelter them from what they need to know and experience. Through trial and error, open communication, unwavering belief, and supportive words and actions, we can teach children the goodness. In all these little ways, you can encourage them to discover their passions, purpose, and path to future personal growth. Can you imagine if someone did that for you when you were younger? Can you imagine if you could move through life without all the baggage of self-doubt and fear childhood can inadvertently put upon us? I, for one, know it would have been easier to work through my mess earlier in life, without pulling others through the mud, as I worked through the messy chapters of my self-discovery. It sounds easy when you think about it, a few slight changes and we could be giving this amazing gift to children. No wrapping required, so save that tape to put other pages of life back together.

Kids Don't Come with Instruction Manuals

Parenting is unique for everyone. My best words to share would be to do what works for you and give yourself lots of grace as we are all human and therefore imperfect. There's no life guidebook. We need to be patient with ourselves and others as we navigate the learning curve. Remember, all humans make mistakes. As a parent of a 12, 10, and 8-year-old, I still have so much to learn. I have so much left to teach my boys, and I know I'll learn even more in the process of trying to do that. Raising future adults is a journey that takes work, dedication, heaps of grace, and loads of love. I have recently come to a point where I can sense how fast it is all going. My oldest only has potentially six more years at home with us, already two-thirds through his time of being under our roof and care. I am now focused on ways to make that last third meaningful, knowing the teenage years will come with a whole new level of parenthood I am not sure I'm prepared for. There will be times of overwhelm, uncertainty, and frustration. When things feel this way, I'll work to pause and consider whatever the basics are that I need to do at that moment, on that day, or during that week. I will remember to start small, get the needs met, and then if I can muster some extras, add them in at that point. I will work to meet my children where they're at and strive to guide them to wherever they need to go. Life is all about learning through each phase as we reach it. Nothing prepares us for all that we face, but with good habits, open communication, and a foundation of support, we can stay afloat in tough times and soar in good times.

It can be easy to lose sight of the immense influence parents, neighbors, relatives, and friends have on kids when we're in the trenches. Small interactions can have big impacts. We need to show kids unconditional love and serve as an example of respect and kindness. If I'm being honest, there are a few adults who would benefit from a refresher course on some of these basics too. Perhaps some of my musings may resonate with you.

Raising The Next Generation of Helpers

At what point did our priorities for profession take precedence over our priority for people? At what point did we start teaching our children that is important to have a goal of being a famous athlete, actor, or other high-status position? Where did the days go when instead of pay, we focused on purpose? Let's turn back a few pages and get back to that, shall we?

If we want to experience success, we need to cultivate the growth of our children as we would a garden. Everything grows with love, consistent work, and intentional effort. Our children are the seeds, and we must plant them in this world with great care. We need to continue to provide the right amount of water and sunlight to help them grow. What traits do we want to cultivate? **Success is not measured by the positions, power, or pay you receive, but instead by the passion, purpose, and people you fill life with.**

Let's teach our kids to grow up with a strong moral character. Let's raise them to know it is their job in life to contribute to something good. Here's what I would love to see on every job description in the future. These skills should not be optional; they should be required:

- Open communication
- Authentic connection
- Kindness
- Humility
- Patience
- Integrity
- Self-reliance
- Respect for self and others
- Positive attitude
- Growth mindset
- Willpower
- Perseverance
- Accountability
- Moral character

I realize this seems like a laundry list of skills, and it won't wash itself. So, let's iron out the reasons these are missing and find a way to get them back into the core of our future success. Some people call these soft skills, but they can be the hardest ones to train in an adult. Soft skills are so valuable in having a productive, effective, and supportive working environment. For example, there are all sorts of instruction manuals and videos to teach tasks, but without tenacity, a new employee may not push on to succeed at learning those tasks. It's good to model these qualities to encourage the building of these traits early in life.

Fend For Yourself

I think part of it is that in too many ways we've started to do our kids' laundry. By showing our love and support only through acts of service, we can keep children from learning to do things for themselves. You know that saying about teaching someone to fish, right? Well, have we stopped teaching our kids what matters; to go out into the ocean and swim on their own? I'm not saying we've been teaching them nothing, but perhaps part of what's broken is we've gotten away from what matters most. We've gotten distracted by trying to do what we think we should be doing for them and have neglected to remember to do what is necessary. When we get caught up in the "shoulds" of life we lose sight of what matters. When we act out of obligation instead of out of what we know is best, important things get overlooked.

I'm not saying throw children to the wolves. We're not animals after all! Be there with loving words of encouragement and support. You need to be there to support them as they fall and get back up. You need to be there to guide them as they learn. However, you can't do everything for them. We need to encourage kids to learn important life skills in order to help them find their own success in life. In the end, they are walking their own path. You can walk beside them, but you can't walk *for* them. That's their job. A job worth doing is worth doing well! Yes, sometimes a job requires tools, and our job is to give kids the tools and make sure they know how to use them. So, where do we start?

The Tools of Life

Let's get back to teaching kids life skills. In the past, kids would contribute to activities associated with hunting and gathering. They worked soil alongside their families to provide for their household. With modern advancements and the introduction of new technologies, many families have lost touch with what's at the root of these life skills. These days, the most activity many kids do with their hands is play video games or type on cellphones or computers. This makes me sad and brings me to the conversation of tools versus toys. We've all likely heard the saying toys are for playing with and tools are for a purpose; not to be played with. Over time we have sheltered our kids from learning to use so many tools for fear they'd hurt themselves or others. Let's bring back their purpose!

This may ruffle some feathers, so I will keep it short and sweet. Instead of teaching kids to fear fire, table saws, knives, guns, and hot stoves; teach them to respect the tool and its intended purpose. It all goes back to education and awareness. We teach kids what to avoid and be afraid of too often, instead of teaching them to be safe, to think, to know the danger, and to respect it, not fear it. To make smart choices, they need to be informed. Why do we teach our kids in ways that don't serve them to live in the real world? We can do better. Again, it's about going back to communication. The same goes for many other objects or experiences we have become accustomed to protecting our kids from. By sheltering them, we are setting them up to enter the world unprepared. They need to know how to use tools with the care and for the purpose intended. They also need to know how to spot true dangers. Pretty simple when you think about it.

Respect and Safety

Some of this should go without saying, but over time, we've abridged our communication too much. Yes, sometimes less is more, but other times we need to add more words of value. As kids grow up, we need to be intentional with our communication. Too often, we throw out words like "stop that," "don't do that," "no," "don't touch that," and other common phrases. This language communicates what not to do. Instead, consider using language that tells them what you want them to do. Also, how often do you use these words out of frustration, impatience, or fear?

Let's think about how we can use our words to help our children understand their actions and the why behind a "no." By doing this they will better understand the reason we want them to take a different action. Let's check ourselves to make sure we're saying those words when it matters. Let's not limit our kids' actions and behavior unless it's warranted. If your kid is climbing high on a playground structure, or up a tree, consider instead of saying any of the above to perhaps offer more useful words.

When my boys started climbing trees, I offered them a guideline for safety that if the limb is smaller than their leg it is not likely strong enough to support them. Offering advice and tips on how to evaluate safety is better than telling them no. Have a conversation, and then, going forward, you can say things like "Does that feel safe?" This language change will encourage them to use their own judgment to decipher if an action is wise to take. Of course, we need to be age appropriate. As kids get older, it's important to let them explore, learn, and make choices for themselves. So much of what we learn is through trial and error with limits.

Feel Your Feelings

It is important that we provide children with the tools and awareness to identify, process, and express their feelings. Instead of allowing emotions to build up over the color of their crayon or the crust not being cut off the bread, we can foster stronger communication. Then, when they become teenagers, we've demonstrated that we can be someone they can feel safe coming to with the hard feelings tied to things like heartbreak, peer pressure, or depression.

If you start to notice yourself thinking your child is being dramatic, too sensitive, needy, or attention-seeking, and you want to give them a punishment or consequence for that behavior, consider instead that they are likely asking for help. It can be hard to verbalize our feelings and needs and throwing tantrums or objects, having meltdowns, crying, and whining may be the only way they know how to communicate. These behaviors are caused by an underlying feeling, a deeper emotion they need help to understand and process.

As adults, we can acknowledge and recognize the cause, not the symptom, and respond to that. By asking questions and responding with compassion, we can teach them it is okay to have feelings, and we can work to show them how to manage their feelings. If we simply tell them to stop doing whatever they are doing, send them to timeout, or reprimand them for the disturbance, they will learn to silence their feelings. They will learn that we are not safe entities to communicate their feelings to, and they may instead feel the need to bury those feelings and deal with them alone in their room, in their chair, or in the corner.

Feelings can be hard to explain at times but finding healthy ways to process and express our feelings is important. **Sometimes it is helpful to think of ourselves like a balloon filled with feelings. If we try to hold in our emotions when we feel sad, mad, scared, or any other heavy feeling, it adds pressure, and we can only hold so many emotions in before we pop.** So, when we experience difficult feelings, it is natural and healthy to stay open and allow emotions to pass through us like the air we breathe.

Let's normalize and make children comfortable knowing that it's okay to feel both hopeful and stressed. They might feel determined one moment and overwhelmed the next. All feelings are okay and normal. It's good for us to feel them and then find ways to move forward and not let heavy feelings keep us down. We can reinforce and explain to them that we are not our feelings. We just experience them. Anger, sadness, hate, depression, fear; this is the rain we sometimes walk in, but we don't become the rain. We know the rain will pass. We walk on and remember the soft glow of the sun will come again. **When we are in the middle of these stormy feelings, it is important we don't send lightning striking at anyone else.** So, it's important and okay to feel stormy feelings, but when we are feeling hurt, it is not okay to use our words or actions to hurt someone else. Having feelings of all types is what makes us human, and important we don't filter them out.

It's great if we can find opportunities to model identifying, processing, and working through feelings with kids. Here's what that might look or sound like. After a few emotional outbursts by my boys one evening, a normal day raising kids, I chose to start a conversation with them at dinner and expressed that I was feeling anxious. I said my chest felt kind of tight, my breathing felt shallow, and I was a bit irritable. I asked if any of them had ever felt that way. Of course, kids being kids, they made jokes and said no. I calmly stopped them and said I didn't appreciate them making jokes. I told them I wanted everyone in our house to be able to talk about their feelings, and I felt unsafe sharing when they responded in that way. I continued by explaining how it is important we know how to identify our feelings and pay attention to how they make our bodies feel. I explained how we can do a body scan to identify where our feelings may be holding up. I said after dinner I might go exercise or take some time to listen to music to help me feel better. I explained how even as grownups, we have lots of feelings, and if they can learn now to be aware of theirs and work through them, they'll have a more comfortable life.

For readers in the trenches of these beautiful, noise-filled, sometimes messy years of raising future adults, I see you. I know how hard it can be to manage your own feelings while trying to model and guide your rugrats. Keep moving through each day, keep trying, keep getting up and doing it again. It matters and you are doing great, even on days it feels like you aren't. Consider the other hard feelings you can have conversations about, identify how that process can make us feel, and give ideas of how to process or manage negative feelings and how we can work to express or release them in a healthy way.

For too long strength has been pushed as an idea of someone who smiles and suffers in silence. Instead, strength should be shown as someone who is brave enough to talk about what they are feeling and has learned how to process them in a healthy way. I want my boys to grow up knowing they can feel and express all of their feelings. Crying isn't a weakness; it is a brave showing of strength. Strength to be comfortable showing emotions, even the more vulnerable ones. A boy can show more than anger and hardness; he can be strong and show empathy. A boy can be tough and sensitive. Emotions and feelings should not be limited or tied to gender—they are tied to being human. Let's not limit our individual humanity and the opportunity to share life with others!

Be Tough and Kind

Life isn't always sunshine and rainbows. We need to prepare our children for the days when people may pick on them, call them names, or push them down. Teach them how to pick themselves up and believe in themselves. Teach them to do better, as the way we respond to unkindness represents us, not others. Let us demonstrate through our actions and responses how to show compassion and empathy for others. Help them understand we don't have to be friends with everyone, but we do need to show respect and kindness to everyone. This doesn't mean we must simply be nice and accept bullying. It means teaching youth there is no reason to use words that put other people down as that only perpetuates the problem. Explain that it's not only pushing, kicking, or hitting that can hurt others. It can hurt to make jokes at other people's expense, to use sarcasm to belittle or demean others, and it can hurt if we don't use our words to stand up for others. Using our words in these ways is unkind and can be truly hurtful, leaving emotional bruises that can last for an exceptionally long time.

It's interesting that many families tell their kids not to say bad words, but what many consider bad are not the worst ones out there. So, excuse my language for a moment, but if we consider s%&#, f#$%, a$&, and other words to be the main ones kids aren't supposed to say, we need to redefine this. When it comes to acceptable words, there is a difference between *naughty* words and *bad* words. *Naughty words* are those I mentioned that are more subjective in how they are used and often more about the appropriate time, place, and audience. *Bad words* are more about intentions and how they can be used in unkind ways against others. So, if we're teaching bad words, we should be discouraging words like stupid, ugly, idiot, wimp, fat, dork, moron, jerk, and others that have the full purpose to insult or put down. Too often we adults can get caught saying some pretty hurtful things ourselves (most let them slip while driving, if we're being honest). As those words fly, our kids are listening and learning, so speak with care. If you happen to be sitting around the table or a fire pit with friends shooting the breeze and some naughty words fly; relax, they are just words if they don't hurt others as you fire them. Again, it's all about time, place, and audience. Let's teach our kids to use respectful words with their elders—teachers, preachers, and grandma. No matter the time, place, or audience, may we be better aware of those bad words.

Being kind goes beyond words. Actions speak loudly, too. So, working to show and teach our kids how to be kind to people that are different from them, as well as those they share commonalities with. To be inclusive whenever possible and to work to not make others feel left out. It can be tough but learning to have our words and actions align with our intentions and character is a great skill. This includes having our words about someone be the same whether they are in the room with us or not. It is in those tough situations of standing up for the people and things in our life according to what we know to be true that character is formed. Our character should not sway based on our current company. Kids need to learn to stand true to themselves and what they believe, regardless of the company they keep.

No Excuses

I don't believe in excuses. To me, there's no such thing as a good excuse. An excuse shows a lack of trying, a lack of choice and action. Not trying to find a solution or finding a way through whatever scenario you are facing is not a good excuse. As I often explain to my kids, if they spent as much time on coming up with possible solutions as they did excuses, they would find success sooner. We need to work to find a way instead of an excuse.

Excuses also give an impression of not taking accountability for a given action or inaction by placing blame on something or someone else. One thing I say to my kids when they start listing excuses: "we can focus on the struggle, or we can look for success". Life is full of choices, and each choice we make comes with a consequence, good or bad. Sure, it seems easy to just blame away our problems and avoid the work of finding solutions. But in doing that, we don't allow problem-solving skills to develop. By staying consistent and not accepting excuses, we help children learn perseverance and responsibility, how to follow instructions, how to commit to an outcome, and how to be accountable. If we don't nurture these good habits and behaviors, their future schooling, career, relationships, and life will be impacted.

Being accountable and acting with integrity builds character. With repetition and encouragement, the choices they make with their thoughts, words, and actions will create strong qualities which will help them in life. By offering examples to them, we can showcase how to stay true to one's beliefs, principles, and morals without excuses. Excuses can come in situations where perhaps they don't care about the outcome or feel there is no consequence of interest to them. With kids, we need to talk them through some of this. Have discussions about how to take others' feelings into account, how our actions or inaction can affect others, and how we need to behave in more collaborative and less selfish ways. If you're breaking a habit of excuses, keep at it. Challenge their excuses every time as one time of having a breakthrough with behavior isn't an instant fix. Also, be sure to catch them doing the right thing and praise them for their responsibility in being accountable.

Talk About the Birds & The Bees

Let's please not do our kids a disservice by not having honest and age-appropriate conversations with them about sex. I'm not saying we need to go all stick figure crazy showing examples with popup book illustrations. But let's just make sure we send our kids into the world with the information they need to be healthy, happy, safe, and successful in all aspects of their life. It doesn't have to be weird. Okay, it's probably going to be weird at first because we've been conditioned to think it must be. But do these conversations have to be difficult? Let's be real, we all got to be here somehow. There are many ways to go about this, so do what works for your family.

Talking Through Discomfort

Not sure where to start? Here are some examples of age-appropriate ways to talk about sex.

- *Kindergarten – 2nd grade*: Boys and girls have different "private" body parts (they should know correct terms for their genitals). We call them "private" as these are the areas we keep covered with our clothes for privacy and no one other than parents or the doctor when your parents are with you should see them. When two people love each other very much they can choose to make a baby together, and doctors can help to bring the baby into the world.

- *3rd – 4th grade*: Basic explanation of how babies are made and brought into the world, educate using the correct terms for male and female genitals. Share awareness of stranger danger.

- *5th grade into middle school*: Conversations about body changes during puberty and what to expect, talks about peer pressure and family morals beliefs around intimacy and sexual behavior.

- *High School*: More in-depth talks about sex and the risks (pregnancy, sexually transmitted infections, etc.). Reiterate family morals/beliefs around sexual behavior. Talks about practicing safe sex (this doesn't have to mean you are encouraging it, but it's important they have the facts). Conversations about not just physical but the emotional element and harm that can be caused if someone chooses to have sex with the wrong person or at the wrong time. The power of NO—respecting other people's choices and bodies. Standing up for themselves if in a pressured situation. Give them ideas and options to stay safe.

- *College*: They are on their own, so hopefully you've taught them well. Remain open and available if they need you. Ensure they know you are always there for them if anything comes up or if they have questions about or need to talk to someone about.

The more we allow natural parts of life to be kept a mysterious secret, or subject to misinformation on the playground or on the back of a bus, the more they end up causing issues in our lives. Quit hiding the truth. It's not helping anyone. Sure, I hope my kids meet their ideal partner who they love and have a future planned with before choosing to be sexually active, but the reality is I should have talks about it all in case their choices don't align with my hopes. It's a disservice to not talk about important things at home because that's where the most important education should happen. Some things are not best learned in a book, online, or from a classmate. They'll have questions, and you should be there to answer them. It's about more than sex education, it's about teaching the values and real-life reasons to wait for the right person before making the big choice to make love with someone. It is a big decision for anyone to make, and therefore, an important conversation to have and care about.

Healthy Touch and Respect for Every Body

Let's talk more about healthy touch and respecting other people's bodies. Our kids need to learn healthy ways to share, advocate for themselves, and show respect for others when it comes to touch. Human touch is powerful if it's shared and received with good intentions and from a kind and gentle heart! This is CRITICAL, so feel free to read that last bit again. Touch can act as a sign of love, caring, and even friendship. There are so many ways to show love and support for those around us. Sure, it comes in more ways than hugs, but I'll start there as they are my favorite. Hugs come in all shapes and sizes appropriate for whatever level of contact a person feels is right with another person. Not a hugger? Perhaps it's a handshake, a pat on the back, a hand to hold, a kiss on the cheek, or simply sitting closely beside someone. It's wonderful to show examples of hugging friends and family members and how touch can serve as a sign that we care enough to reach out in a more personal way.

Unfortunately, not everyone has good intentions, and we need to make sure kids know the signs of danger. Educate them about the signs of bad touch, not to scare them, but rather because knowledge is power. We all need to be respectful of people's boundaries and personal bubbles. As my kids have gotten older, I have started to ask if they want a hug. If they say yes, I approach with open arms, and if they say no, I respect and honor their words. I explain it is always up to them and their choice, just as it is the choice of others what they are comfortable with. No means no, EVERY TIME!

Whether a hug, a handshake, or any other loving touch, everyone has a right to choose how they share and receive love. So that means if that uncle or aunt comes in for a hug and your child isn't feeling it at that moment, do not force it. Allow them to listen to their bodies and speak up for what feels good and what doesn't. I'm not trying to say that your uncle or aunt is being harmful in sharing their love, but these are moments when you can empower and teach your child that it's okay to say no, it's okay to speak up.

If you happen to be that aunt or uncle, help empower their voice and choice by respecting those boundaries. It may seem like a small gesture for now, but it can have a big effect on their confidence to use their voice in the future. So, please teach and show your kids the power of good, healthy touch, and how to give and receive this kind of love.

Work Before Play

I'm not sure when it happened, but in many homes, kids have an unrealistic expectation of what they "deserve." In modern times kids have all sorts of playtime. Yes, kids should play but at what point did it become normal for the kids' activity schedules to run the house schedule? I'm not saying we should not strive to give our kids life experiences, but I think we've been looking at it wrong.

So, what this means is we're doing a disservice if we fill kids' lives with all that extra stuff and forget the basics. Why have we packed our days full of activities that are not necessary? We've created so many activities to occupy or entertain our kids. Do you remember what amazing things come from being bored? Imagination, dreams, creativity, and learning that they can't always get everything handed to them in a perfectly planned package of fun. Sometimes they have to invent their own fun. Life has gotten so busy with all those other activities we are often not leaving room to teach our kids other important stuff. So, let's step back a moment and consider where the priorities should be. What will most benefit them in the long run? Also, are you building in time for rest? Like adults, they need time to recharge, too, and can suffer from being overscheduled.

They are called extracurricular activities for a reason. EXTRAcurricular means it is an activity that occurs in addition to basic studies. They are not at the core of what is required. Many extracurricular activities are good; they can teach important lessons in leadership, socialization, teamwork, and being part of a community. However, in 2022, it is not uncommon for a child to have activities planned for every day, or to play a sport or sports year-round. If your kid is guaranteed to be a professional athlete, by all means, keep them in three sports a season. But the odds are not in their favor. So, consider cutting back on the extras and get back to the basics.

In place of so many extra activities outside of the house, why not take time for more enriching activities as a family? Teach them how to cook, do laundry, clean up after themselves, help with chores, change a tire, sew, build something with their hands, work in the yard, help a neighbor, or volunteer in their community. We do not have kids simply to serve their every desire while they live in our homes. We have kids so we can share our love with them and raise them to be good humans. If you aren't showing them and teaching them what it takes to be a good human, where do you think they'll learn it?

Teamwork

These days, sports get serious at a much earlier age and the competitive spirit can take hold before the great parts of teamwork are taught. We need to remember to teach our children sometimes you win, and sometimes you learn. In every game, there is always something to learn, and often, our confidence must be set aside to take that opportunity to improve. Yes, it's great to celebrate successes, but it's also important to be humble in our wins. It's important to learn to appreciate the value of the team and how working together brings the biggest opportunity for success. Children must learn to show respect for their opponents whether they win or lose. What are other important things we can teach the next generation through sports? I'll talk more about successful habits and behavior we can show through example in Chapter 8. When they are young, these habits of teamwork and learning from their losses as much from their wins will help build character. These are not exclusive to a sports court or field either, so look for the opportunities to teach these lessons.

Make Time for Fun

Yes, we live busier lives, but must we stop having fun as a family? Perhaps this ended for some around the time people stopped joining around a table to eat a meal? Well, that needs to change. The connection of a family is what drives life and is at the core of all that is good. Family is the essence that helps define our very identity. What may seem like fun and games now are the memories they will hold dear in their hearts as they get older. Don't keep them from all those happy memories because life is busy. Life will always feel busy. Make time for what matters.

Peter Pan had some insight into what makes life good —being silly and having fun with kids. I mean, you don't have to wear tights if you don't want to, but if that brings out the sweet joy of childhood, I say prance around in whatever you've got! If there is something that makes you smile or giggle with pure delight, and if it hurts no one to do so—stop holding yourself back. Kids need to see adults being silly, they need to see us having fun. They learn by watching us. Kids should be kids, they should have fun on their own too, but they enjoy us being a part of their activities sometimes. We know the best things are learned at home. The most important things that create their core are learned within the safe and loving communities they live in with their family and friends. So, never lose the kid inside you and show that carefree feeling. Caring is free and we need to care about the right things. Don't be afraid to get your hands dirty.

More Time Outside

Speaking of dirt, it makes me think of the saying God made dirt, so dirt doesn't hurt. Whether you are religious or not, I think most of us could agree that statement is true. Dirt does not hurt. We need to see more kids out playing in the dirt instead of playing on screens. There are so many benefits to kids playing out in the fresh air and exploring natural areas. Let's not make technological advancements the reason we stay away from the natural beauty and important things nature brings us. Nature has a way of helping us focus on the current experience we are having and relieves some of the weight of life that follows us. We need to ensure our youth stay connected with nature and learn to respect and care for it to reap all the benefits in the future.

A wonderful thing about nature is it does not cost anything. It has no expectations of us, and it doesn't matter what shape or form we are in. Nature accepts you no matter what. If you have a young family, or if you are helping care for young relatives or neighbors and are not sure where to start—look for the resources around you. You're not the first one nervous to head into nature alone or feel lost about where to go, and you don't have to do it alone. There are great resources to help you take that first step into nature*.[4]

---

[4] Resources included at end of book

No matter what season of life you are in, I guarantee there are groups and communities to support you in taking your first step outside. Find a trail, explore a park, or take a walk through the neighborhood. An adventure doesn't have to be anything big, and you don't need any special equipment to get out there. You only need the willingness to step outside the comfort of your home to see the possibilities outside your door. When you stop and look, you'll find growth and beauty abounds. It's all around us. Wherever you live, it's a wonderful day in the neighborhood, so put your shoes on and move one foot in front of the other. Your feet will take you wherever you need to go.

Take Out the Trash

Respecting nature. I don't know if you've noticed, but humans have kind of become slobs. It appears many people these days were born in a barn or something. Okay, not really, as guaranteed if that were the case their parents would have told them to quit being such a pig and to clean up after themselves. Whether you grew up in a city, in the country, or in the middle of the desert—let's all lead by example. If we continue to trash where we live, what is that helping?

Unless we want kids to grow up like Oscar the Grouch living in their own trash can paradise—it's time we do something about it. If we aren't going to work for change, we can't be bothered by the problem. Talking about a problem does no good if no one is working toward a solution. So, roll up your sleeves and get out there to do your part to help clean up the mess we've made. It doesn't matter if you literally made the mess. Didn't your parents teach you that? If not, let's go back to that bit I mentioned about community. It's about more than you or me; we all need to fulfill our piece of the bigger puzzle.

The first step is taking action. The best thing we can do is start to make minor changes each day to make a difference in teaching those around us and doing our part to clean up our mess. The worst thing we can do is nothing. So, take some initiative and start a park clean-up. Plan to take a stroll on the beach and invite your friends to bring some gloves and pick up trash as you walk together. If we look at the mountain of garbage it can be overwhelming, but let's not assume we must climb an entire mountain in a day. Let's start by taking one step of helpful action each day to make a difference where we live, in the places we love, and include those in our life who we know care enough to help. Start by consistently teaching and showing those in our homes and our communities to respect what is outside our doors.

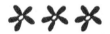

Chapter 4
Just Be Yourself

Of all our relationships, the one we have with ourselves is the most important. By allowing ourselves to be authentic and comfortable in our own skin, we can open ourselves to a happier, healthier, and more successful life. Once we can accept ourselves for who we are, it is easier to accept and connect with others. Once we learn and acknowledge what we like, want, and need in life, we can seek others who have common and mutual interests. We can enrich our lives with relationships that add to our experience in life. Although we need to have a strong relationship with ourselves, life is not meant to spend alone. Although we are all different, we are the same in so many ways. A community can help us feel a sense of belonging and mutual understanding. By joining and sharing with others, we will find more happiness, support, and togetherness.

The path to a good life is paved with truth, love, and kindness. I appreciate people who are comfortable enough to share their hearts, stories, and struggles in life with those they care about. It's not always easy to be vulnerable with ourselves or others. However, I feel once you can find the courage to come out from behind that mask of keeping up appearances and let your real self show, it lifts such a weight from wherever you are carrying it. Life is meant to be shared, even the messy parts. You are not alone, and I for one am not judging you for the parts of your life that carry hurt. Want to know a secret? We all have them; it's part of being human.

If you find yourself having to tiptoe around others, you're not walking among the right people. May we all find confidence in being ourselves without apology or judgment, without others making us feel we're doing it wrong, and without the pressure to be something or someone we're not. Never question whether you're enough or too much—for those who love you, you are just right, as you are! So, let's choose to walk alongside those who love us for all that we are. Find comfort in those who show empathy, understanding, and genuine caring. Spend time with people who make you feel good about yourself, who don't make you feel the need to question what they say about you when you are not with them. Be in relationship with people who lift you up rather than push you down. Don't accept less than what you need from those in your circle of life!

Sometimes you have to redraw that circle, bring it in, or draw it out to include those who fit best in your life and will dance through life with you instead of tiptoeing. Know who your people are and let's also do our best to be those people for others!

Vulnerability

When we don't talk about what is going on in our lives, when we hold back from sharing life with each other, we do a disservice to our relationships. Has it become the norm to default to small talk? I hope not in all circles of life. Richer are the days when we can talk about real life and learn about the people we spend our time with. The next time you cross paths with a friend or family member and they say, "Hi, how are you?" Don't say "I'm fine," "can't complain," or "good!" Open your mouth and say how you feel and what you're thinking. Talk about what's happened in your day. If it's a friend or family member, they will want to know all of it. They will want to hear about how your morning started with your dog puking all over the floor and then you spilled coffee on yourself trying to rush out the door as you were running late again. They will want to hear you had an enjoyable conversation with an old friend, or that you're excited to be planning your next vacation. People care.

If you've mastered what I mentioned about thoughts, words, and interpretation—there is not much to fear in opening up to people. Of course, being authentic is tied to trust. How much of ourselves we share can depend on how safe we feel with that person or in that situation. I'm not encouraging fakeness, but we do have to protect our vulnerability to a point and choose how many details we share with whom. The more we can communicate with kindness, openness, and without filters or shutting our thoughts or heart down, the freer we will feel. It is damaging to constantly hold things in or feign strength simply to impress others. Eventually, after hiding so many pieces of yourself you will begin to feel lonely, resentful, and like no one sees you, appreciates you, or values your presence. Guess what, in a way, you did that to yourself! I've been there. This is exactly what I used to do—just business, nothing personal, and keep smiling. Well, that wasn't cutting it. So I decided to step out of my comfort zone and share more of my words and heart. I started to show the real me, and I did not always smile through it. Was it scary? You bet your bottom dollar! Do you know what happened though? Once I started telling the truth and sharing more of myself, I got a great return on that investment. I got to feel supported by others, who, once the sharing started, also began sharing what was a struggle or a celebration in their life. I felt like I wasn't alone or crazy anymore. I began to realize we all have a messy, scary, out of control, or painful part of our life that others can't see just looking in.

When we become more open, we can more clearly recognize each other's humanity. This is how our empathy and compassion can grow. We must have the courage to take off that mask of insecurity, shame, guilt, and feelings of not enough. **Feelings of shame and self-doubt shrivel away when you share your story in safe places.** Once you can allow that vulnerability to peek through, it can be so refreshing! I can't take all the credit for this revelation. Looking back, it was a few strong friends in my life that had opened my heart to this and helped me break down those barriers. I will forever be thankful to the people who crossed my path and pushed me to be more open and just be myself, that I was enough.

Why do we assume people don't want to know more? What's the point of all the talking if by the end of the day I couldn't tell you anything of value about you from our conversations? I value you; I care about your life, and I appreciate knowing more because I care. Assume other people feel the same way. You may be a stranger to me, but I can say without a doubt in my heart I do care about your life and all the joy and mess within it. It matters; share it with others!

Take Off the Mask

Letting the raw and authentic version of ourselves show can be scary at first. It can be intimidating to let those imperfect and vulnerable parts of life start peeking out from behind the curtain of what we think we should let others see. Self-doubt and fear want to take over. When I struggled to juggle work and family life and felt I was losing myself in the late nights of burning the candle at both ends; I kept smiling through it. On the inside, I was buried in stress from trying to build my business, raise my boys, manage the house, attend to my husband's needs, be an active community member, and in the process, I lost sight of myself. I didn't talk to anyone about how I was struggling. I figured that was the way it was supposed to be, so I powered on. I remember people commenting on how I seemed to have it all together, how they didn't know how I juggled it all, how I was such a good Mom and wife, and how I always seemed so happy. The thing is, life is a juggling act, and those looking in may see some perspective of magic looking in from the outside. When that happens, we can feel the need to keep measuring up to those expectations; those ridiculous expectations of what life should look like. I took those compliments and felt proud at first. As the years went on and I kept trying to be perfect—I started to feel like a fake.

You see, in those early days of building my business and raising kids and figuring out married life, most of my days were spent cleaning up other people's messes. I had to prepare healthy meals for the family and make sure there were clean clothes to wear. I tried to plan fun outings to enrich our lives, and I tried to find a community of other families to connect and share life with. My life was filled with so many busy days of running around while also feeling I'd accomplished nothing. On weekdays, I'd try to sneak in some work time if I happened to magically get the kids to nap at the same time. By the time my husband got home from work, it was time to prepare dinner and that's when my work shift change began. I would retreat to my office and lock the door for my precious work hours, and often I would not come back out until everyone was asleep. If I happened to come down early my husband would usually be relaxing by the television. If it was late, or if he happened to fall asleep with the kids, I'd come down to a quiet house. I'd often come down from my office and find messes from dinner still at the table or cluttering the kitchen counter. I'd start in on cleaning up the kitchen and the husband would ask why I couldn't relax and sit down with him. I'd want to sit for a moment to relax and unwind, and then notice the loads of clean laundry I managed to get through during the day still in the living room, waiting for *someone* to fold them; finishing up dinner and bedtime routines surely kept my husband busy while I was working, so I figured that *someone* was me.

During those years, I acknowledged my husband had a full day of work and enjoyed relaxing by watching television at night. I knew his days were filled with stress but found myself feeling resentful that he hadn't thought to clean up after dinner or fold laundry while he watched television. I felt this but never communicated it. I assumed since I stayed home with the kids during the day (while also running my business), I was responsible for the management of the home. So I would continue with the chores of family life before sitting down. I knew the shift change routine was hard on my husband and at times felt like he resented me working as he missed time with me. I tried to dedicate some nights to spending time with him watching a show after getting the kids tucked in and ignoring the chores. I would stay up with him until he went to sleep and then I would try to get in a few hours of work. That routine was not sustainable, and as I got more clients, those nights on the couch were fewer.

This was a lonely time in my life. I felt tired, overwhelmed, unseen, and unappreciated. I loved being home with my boys and would not change that for anything, but it came with feelings of guilt I hadn't expected. The juggling of mom and businesswoman during the day was difficult. When I had a deadline or urgent work task, I felt guilty if I had to address it while my boys were awake. If I was busy with the boys and didn't respond as quickly to communications from my clients, I felt bad for my delay in follow-up. On top of the mom/businesswoman juggling act, I also assumed the responsibility of trying to ensure I kept my husband happy. I began to realize if I shared details about fun things I did with the boys during the day, my husband would make comments that he wished he could've done that with them, or how that sounded like more fun than his day at work. I began to feel bad for sharing these happy moments with him, so began to tell him less and less so as not to make him feel bad for missing out. So instead, when he would come home and share things that were a struggle at work, instead of sharing the good things the boys and I had done, I started sharing the struggles. This became a negative cycle. I was filtering my life into what I could share with him and what I felt I shouldn't. I started looking elsewhere for people I could share all parts of my life with. I created a whole community of friends outside my family that filled this area of support and communication.

I missed having conversations with other grownups and being able to talk to people about the highs and lows of parenting young kids. I wanted to share moments of success with my business too and the frustrations of managing to work from home while raising kids, but in my friend circle, there weren't many that could connect or relate. At times, I worried my husband felt resentful or jealous of me for starting the business. He had always dreamed of owning a business, so I didn't talk business with him often. It was a mutual choice for me to stay home and raise the kids, and it just so happened that I found a way to do both. I chose to continue working once we had kids because it brought me a sense of accomplishment and fulfillment. I loved being a mom, but I also liked feeling I could support myself. It was a struggle to do both, but I do not regret it.

By keeping to small talk, avoiding conflict, and not talking about everything that was going on and how it made us FEEL, my husband and I were both building up assumptions about what the other was thinking or feeling. We were building walls that broke our communication with one another. If you are in a loop of trying to put on a face of perfection or trying to live up to unrealistic expectations, stop and consider: who is setting these magic expectations? Most likely, it's you. You may be allowing a few around you to feed into your thoughts and unrealistic expectations, or more likely, making assumptions about what they expect of you. Set your own expectations, know your value, and accept nothing less!

We've probably all heard the phrase, "fake it until you make it," and that may work for some, but I say, **"be real while you heal."** Faking it through life and attempting perfection will only hurt you in the long run. Sometimes by acknowledging what we're struggling with or challenged by, we can start taking steps to improve our lives. We each have the power to write our own story, so heal what is hurting you, talk through the problems, and work to make the future chapters of your life good. I love an idea I heard on a podcast by Brené Brown*[5] about choosing discomfort over resentment. By taking a few minutes to bring up a conversation that makes you uncomfortable, you can avoid years of resentment. Face your feelings, your problems, and those hard conversations. Exhale and move forward. No faking it required.

Love The Skin You're In

This one gets me a little fired up. Body insecurity and body shaming are big issues in our society. I have struggled with body insecurity and body shaming throughout my life, and at one point, it hit rock bottom. My wellness was negatively affected by skipping meals and other poor eating habits. Society teaches us that a smaller waistline is a positive thing. The truth is, even when I was the thinnest I'd ever been in my adult life, I still wasn't happy with my body. Then, I was diagnosed with something that will require me to be on medication for the rest of my life, and the side effects mess with my metabolism, causing increased appetite, and therefore, weight gain. I've already started to see the effects of it, and like other times in life, I've been tempted to feel betrayed and disappointed by my body. When the bullies in my brain start telling me these things, it's a reminder that I have to continue to work to change my mindset and relationship with food and my body image.

When does our conception of body image start? When we are young! As a girl, I developed early, and boys gave me attention on the playground, walking the halls at school, and friendly gatherings outside of school. I remember feeling uncomfortable with the attention I received. One memory especially sticks with me. At one point, I wore a shirt that had a modest, small heart cut out in the front and someone called me a slut for wearing it. They said I was trying to get attention from boys. Those words hurt; I just thought it was a cute top. I remember feeling embarrassed and ashamed. Over time I started to change how I dressed. I would wear more baggy clothes and less fitted outfits to avoid drawing attention to my developing figure. Even in college, I tended to wear baggy clothes so as not to accentuate my curves. Some would joke that I dressed like a boy.

---

[5] Resources included at end of book

In high school, I felt pressured to look a certain way. Despite wearing loose clothing, I wanted to be thin. I would restrict my eating or skip meals altogether in an attempt to control my weight. Thankfully, I was never able to make myself throw up, although not for lack of trying. I was already starting a cycle of poor self-image and unhealthy habits. In college, someone I cared about called me beefy. They said they were trying to say I was strong, but what I heard was them calling me fat. Another time, someone told me if I ever got too heavy, they would tie me up behind a car and let me run. Although they said it was a joke, it still made me wonder if they were insinuating that I was already too heavy. It made me feel uncared for. That's the thing with jokes, they often have some truth in them and when said to someone else as the butt of the joke—it's not so funny. I also have countless memories of walking beside someone and hearing them make comments about how women were dressed or about their weight. Comments like, "She really shouldn't be wearing those pants."; or "doesn't she have friends to tell her not to wear things like that?" Sure, these comments weren't directed at me, but they could have been. I heard that judgment and criticalness and started to think others must be thinking about me this way too. When we already feel insecure even well-intentioned comments can be received as criticism.

I know there are versions of this story shared by many. As technology becomes more advanced, our insecurities can be exacerbated. We can be pulled into thinking we have to filter out the imperfect parts of ourselves. Click a button and it softens your skin tone, removes blemishes, smooths out wrinkles, and accentuates your features. Enough clicks and you may start to not recognize yourself, or worse yet, you may start to wish you looked like this unrealistic picture. No one is perfect, and that's what makes life beautiful. So, I am sending you confidence, courage, hope, and self-acceptance. I am working on manifesting these for myself as well. There's nothing wrong with showing your true colors, blemishes, and every human detail. Be yourself. You are amazing the way you are! And it isn't just ladies, I know guys have their own set of body insecurities and pressures too. I won't pretend to assume to know how that feels, but both men and women can be their own worst critics. Over the years, women often carry the pressure of worrying about the freshman 15, trying to attract a mate, being able to get pregnant and grow a healthy baby, being able to breastfeed, and losing baby weight. Many of these things are not in our control, and we can feel betrayed or disappointed by our bodies for not measuring up.

The first time I felt betrayed by my body was when I had a miscarriage. It was my first pregnancy, and I was between 11 and 12 weeks when I lost the baby. I felt so helpless and incredibly discouraged. I was certain I had done something wrong or hadn't done something right causing it to happen. I was heartbroken for the future I thought I had. There were so many questions. And to add insult to injury, my body needed help to complete the process. I required a medical procedure to complete the miscarriage. It was painful and it felt endless to get through it all. My body had failed me. It is hard to have our body do things we don't understand and can't control.

We often build expectations around what is acceptable and attractive in society, in our friend groups, through our churches, and in our families regarding our bodies. These expectations are often built by other people, not ourselves. If we're a little fluffy or curvy, we are expected to wear baggy clothing, nothing too tight or revealing. As we get older, we are told we can't dress a certain way as it is too youthful. Women are told to be modest and cover their bodies or fear being seen as inviting trouble. With all these voices, messages, and expectations how do we build confidence and comfort around our bodies to battle the shame?

Most other people see our physical appearance and abilities in a more favorable and less judgmental light than we do. In the end, holistic health is key! Holistic health involves looking at many dimensions of our wellness. It focuses on the whole person—physical, mental, emotional, social, intellectual, and spiritual. In all these areas, it is about progress, not perfection. To attain balance and wellness in life, we must focus on our whole person. It takes time to change how we see ourselves. We must work to support our wellness (not thinness) every day. Our weight will ebb and flow, so don't measure your beauty by that standard. Each laugh line, grey hair, or stretch mark is a part of your story, but they don't define you. Let's toss those judgments, filters, and unrealistic expectations in the trash. Let's choose to change our language around beauty and how we measure it for ourselves. Every single body on Earth is beautiful. No matter the shape, size, color, or orientation—every body is beautiful, unique, and worthy of love and respect. No one should feel ashamed of their own flesh and bones.

What do we get from putting ourselves or others down? Each time we are tempted to complain about a part of our body, let's instead find a way to compliment one of our strengths. We are inadvertently teaching the next generation through our language and example. If enough people care, we can hopefully change the toxic body culture for our kids. Time to fight back those bullies in our brains telling us we're not good enough! Let's do better! What part of your body can you celebrate today?

Each person's level of body modesty is a personal choice. If someone chooses to cover up, it doesn't mean they are not proud of their body or restricting themselves. If someone chooses to cover less, it doesn't mean they are doing it for attention, being scandalous, or inappropriate. I wish we all could allow others to live according to their own choice and comfort and not require them to comply with preset expectations or fear of judgment. That's what makes life so colorful and interesting—choice.

Great pep talk, huh? But what comes next? Do we keep moving forward in this unhealthy cycle? If we know the body culture that is being promoted is not serving us in healthy ways, let's quit buying into it and promoting it in our language and actions. Let's stop putting so much value into the thought that our bodies determine our personal identities; that we have to fit into some norm of what physical attractiveness is supposed to be or look like. Let's quit making ourselves and others feel bad about who they are based on their appearance. Imagine how vastly different we would see each other if our eyes saw souls instead of bodies, and how much more beautiful our interactions in this world could be. A great first step is considering how I talk to myself about my own body; if I wouldn't say it to a friend, I should not say it to myself. I encourage you to practice doing the same.

Quit Faking It – Life Isn't Perfect

Life is messy, but that's not new. What is new is that we are all trying to hide our messes and only show a picture-perfect version of our lives. By doing this we are holding back our true potential which is much greater than whatever we're pretending to be! No one's life is picture-perfect and when we live our lives trying to frame it that way, we build walls of insecurity around ourselves. We worry we may slip up and someone will see through us. Can you imagine the weight that would be lifted if you weren't afraid to let it all hang out? Hold on, keep your pants on... I'm not talking about those parts. Let's keep sharing at a PG level in crowds as we still have to keep some level of privacy and order in our larger community. However, if you have a close group of neighbors or friends, why not open up and share more of your heart and struggles.

For 15 years I tried to put on the face of the 1950's "perfect" wife and mother. I was the world's best trier. I rarely shared when I was having struggles with my kids out of a fear that people would judge me and be critical of my parenting. When I struggled in my marriage, I did not talk about it as I thought it reflected poorly on how I was not measuring up as a wife. When the business in the bedroom needed a new business plan, I felt shame in talking about such sensitive subjects with people. Some of us are taught that these are the things we should not speak of. Guess what, there's no book telling us how to live our lives. We have to learn and teach ourselves as we go. To ease the feelings of isolation and self-doubt, talk it out!

The truth is, we can't heal if we keep pretending we're not hurt. The more ownership we have over our lives, the less out of control we will feel. When we own our failures, we can find opportunities for improvement. When we own our successes, we can celebrate. So don't let your failures get you down. Failure is an opportunity to grow. I recently realized we had taught our kids a poor example of striving for perfection. So now we're having those hard conversations trying to unteach what they learned and allow ourselves to be vulnerable and admit to our imperfections. Today I focus on sharing how we strive for progress and learn from our mistakes. I am talking about knowing when and how to ask for help. New examples, new learning, new growth for the whole family. Grace and compassion for our imperfect and beautiful parts is key. Not being too proud to admit when you need help is huge!

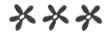

words to grow by

"Growth begins when we begin to accept our own weaknesses"

Jean Vanier

"Turn your wounds into wisdom."

Oprah Winfrey

"All change is not growth, as all movement is not forward."

Ellen Glasgow

"Without continual growth and progress, such words as improvement, achievement, and success have no meaning."

Benjamin Franklin

"It always seems impossible until it's done."

Nelson Mandela

Chapter 5
Life's Roadblocks and Detours

Remember life is a journey, not a destination, and sometimes the track we thought we were on (personally, professionally, or otherwise) gets derailed, and it can be easy to spiral into the should've, could've, and would've thoughts. When this happens, I try to remember I am still the driver. The place I am at right now is not my destination, it is only a part of the journey. Through each twist and turn on this journey, I can choose to take my foot off the gas for a bit, slow down, and focus on where I am in that moment. I may not know what is around the curve ahead. I can acknowledge I don't have control over each roadblock, detour, or derailing. I can appreciate that I do have control over whether I keep driving with the pedal to the metal. I can choose to pull off for a moment and reassess the map I am following. Maybe I need to add in a few rest stops to my journey. A big part of life is taking time to embrace the journey and letting go of things we can't control. So tomorrow, perhaps you'll choose to drive with the windows down and your favorite music turned up, maybe you'll choose to take the scenic route with the best view, maybe you'll just enjoy the drive.

Each day brings new challenges and we will continue to feel both joy and sorrow. Life will never be perfect; it wasn't built that way. Every challenge and every joy and every sorrow-filled moment helps to build our life story. Through the ups and downs, we feel the variety that life offers. Embrace it, learn from it, enrich your life with relationships built from it. Feel the sorrow, and then let go of it knowing what you have learned in the darkness will light your path forward. Continue to share with others. Life is tough, but so are you. So let your strength and light shine brightest, especially on hard days as that's when we need to feel our light the most. **Once you learn how to start calling yourself out on the crap that is holding you back, you can use it as fertilizer for growth**. First, you have to acknowledge what you continue to stumble on.

Growth Tool

Be Done With It – Fertilizer for Growth!

What areas of your life are holding you back from your potential for health, happiness, and success? When I think of personal growth I consider there are two key parts.

1. Taking action to add things to life that bring us better health and happiness.
2. Choosing to be done with things that no longer serve us or bring good energy to our lives.

What do you need to move forward with and what do you need to be done with? Below are some examples of mine, perhaps they can be a starting point to help you dig in and identify yours. Write yours down and reference them often so you can continue to align with your intentions and goals.

- I am done worrying whether people like me and instead focus on liking myself.
- I am done over apologizing and taking blame for things that are not my fault.
- I am done comparing myself to others and feeling I am not enough.

- I am done allowing others' negative energy to permeate my heart.
- I am done overthinking the past, and instead, am focused on the now and the future.
- I am done pouring love and attention into people who don't reciprocate.
- I am done judging and shaming myself for past mistakes.
- I am done trying to prove myself to anybody.
- I am done holding unrealistic ideals and expectations of life.
- I am done feeling embarrassed by my tendencies to sing, dance, and be silly.
- I am done trying to change for others.
- I am done being anything other than my authentic self.

We may not be able to change the world, but we can change how we experience and interact in it.

Ending the Shame Cycle

I had a big aha moment recently when reading the book, *"I Thought it Was Just Me (but it isn't): Making the Journey From "What Will People Think?" to "I Am Enough."* written by Brené Brown. It's a great read that goes deeper into topics of shame, guilt, embarrassment, humiliation, problems with perfectionism, and being authentic. I had not thought too much about the concepts of shame vs guilt in the past. Growing up in a church community and attending private Catholic school as a young girl, I became familiar with what I knew of as "Catholic guilt". I became a "bad Catholic" as I grew up and apart from the religious structures of the church. In my mind, I was no longer a good Catholic girl because I didn't attend church every Sunday, in fact I barely attended church at all. I attributed that for making me feel bad about myself and my choices. Ends up shame is more on point for the feelings and judgements I felt. For me it didn't end at just church attendance. Feeling shameful was something I applied to multiple areas in my life. Realizing that was a turning point.

Consider how you internalize your thoughts and feelings around mistakes or bad decisions. Are you imposing shame on yourself or guilt? Here's how to know the difference. Shame is thinking, "I am a failure". Guilt is thinking "I have failed at this task". Guilt can actually be a positive motivator of change, while shame typically leads to worse behavior or paralysis. Are you someone that after forgetting to text your friend on their birthday thinks, I am a bad friend? Or instead, do you focus on the specific choice or task and perhaps choose to put a reminder on your calendar to remember next time? Consider how you communicate with yourself and others and which message you are supporting. When we allow ourselves to not personalize the experience or action, we can instead focus on the behavior and see the opportunity for learning and improvement. If we make it personal it can insinuate it is a character flaw, and we can at times put ourselves and others into a corner of creating a self-fulfilling prophecy. A message that does not encourage change, learning, or growth.

Shame is a very painful emotion and you may even know how your body physically responds to this emotion. People are typically prone to either a guilt response or a shame response, but we each can change that mindset. The antidote (so to speak) for shame is empathy. If we are in a mindset of judgment, stereotyping, or thinking we are superior or better than others (or the reverse, feeling we are not good enough) it creates a disconnect. Often this mindset is rooted in fear, insecurity, unrealistic expectations, or our own shame. When we can instead open our hearts and minds to compassion, empathy, and authentic connection we can allow for our skills in resilience and humanity to grow, which in turn relieves others' feelings of shame.

What is eye-opening is to realize shame starts early. As parents, aunts, uncles, friends, teachers, coaches, and involved community members, we have the opportunity to raise children who are compassionate, resilient, kind, and authentic. We can use our language and actions to communicate without using shame, without falling prey to holding others to unrealistic expectations or stereotypes. It starts with us and our ability to dig in and start learning about the way shame shows up in our lives. By healing ourselves we then empower those in our circle of influence by not hurting them in the same ways.

Spiritual Care – Walking in Faith

In case you are on a journey in spiritual care and identity I want to share a bit about where I am on my journey to spiritual health. I have struggled with my religious identity for years. After high school when I stopped going to church regularly—I had a disconnect from organized religion. I never stopped having faith or believing in a higher power, but suddenly when I found myself in conversations and people asked what church I went to, I had an overwhelming feeling of shame. This has taken some soul searching and work to open my perspective to how I interpret my faith and spirituality. These days I am getting more comfortable when people ask that I say I attend the church of nature and life. I believe in the teachings of love, compassion, kindness, pursuit of learning, and growth. I am not a bad person for not attending or raising my children in a church. What would be bad is not living and raising my kids according to what is good, regardless of where I sit on a Sunday morning. I believe in something bigger than myself, a greater energy or spirit.

Shame holds us back from growth so it's important that we stay humble to the mystery of faith as that is what gives us the language of journey, change, and transformation. Whether in a church, on a trail, around a table sharing a meal with friends or family, or any place where you feel an energy of hope and promise. Spend time there. Release yourself from the expectations of what faith or spirituality is supposed to look like. There are many interpretations in this world and none are absolute, aside from what you feel in your heart. There is not a box that you need to fit within when it comes to your spirituality, so be mindful and kind to yourself.

Practice Self-Compassion

Whatever path you are on, you are bound to run into moments of self-doubt, fear, and worry. At some turns, you may fall into the shadows of shame, embarrassment, or guilt. We are all imperfect and flawed humans, and our thoughts can get the best of us in times when we fail or make mistakes. Make sure you take steps to stand up to those bullies in your brain causing negative thoughts to spiral and prove them wrong. Show yourself some self-compassion. That's right, when you find yourself in these hurtful thought patterns, consider for a moment- would you ever talk to a friend that way? We are our own worst critics. Empathy and compassion for others is one thing, even harder is offering that grace and acceptance to ourselves.

Standing Up to the Those Bullies in our Brains

We must be careful with our thoughts as they are the hinge point for so many things in our lives. When we allow ourselves to believe irrational and inaccurate thoughts it can lead to so many problems and issues in all aspects of our life. When you give power to the bullies in your brain, your thoughts can deceive you and lead you to believe things that aren't true. These bullies can push you around, kick you down, and cause feelings of inadequacy, shame, guilt, and bad feelings. So, take a moment to look around that playground inside your brain and figure out who's playing nice. Stick with the friendly and good thoughts and leave those negative nellies to play alone.

Identify Your Bullies

So how do you tell the difference between a friend and an enemy when it's all in your head? Below are some examples of common bullies, perhaps you'll identify ones you struggle with and then learn how to stand up to them.

- **All-or-Nothing Thinking**: Seeing things as black and white, good and bad, success or failure without any gray area.
- **Overgeneralizing**: Taking an incident and generalizing it to the rest of life, often plagued with words like always, never, everyone, no one, everything, nothing.
- **Filtering out the Positive**: Focusing on the one bad thing or mistake instead of the seven good things or successes.
- **Mind Reading**: Assuming you know what others are thinking, feeling, or what their intentions are.

- **Catastrophizing**: Assuming bad outcomes or jumping to expect worse case scenarios.
- **Emotional Reasoning**: When we are so strongly influenced by our emotions that we assume they indicate objective truth and don't consider there is a need for supporting facts of evidence. Often attributed to negative emotions
- **Labeling**: Labeling people and experiences based on isolated incidents.
- **Fortune Telling**: Jumping to conclusions and predicting doom and gloom instead of considering other possible outcomes.
- **Personalization**: Assuming situations and experiences revolve around us which leads to taking everything personally.
- **Unreal Ideal**: Unfairly comparing ourselves to others or unrealistic expectations.

Overthinkers Not So Anonymous

"Hold on. Let me overthink this." Do you find yourself spiraling in thoughts like this?

- Dwelling on past events or situations
- Second-guessing decisions you've made
- Replaying your mistakes in your mind
- Rehashing challenging or uncomfortable conversations
- Fixating on things you can't control, change, or improve
- Imagining the worst-case scenario or outcome
- Following your worries out of the present moment and into an unchangeable past or unforeseeable future
- "Running your list" while trying to fall asleep
- Questioning but never making a decision or taking action

If this sounds like you, you may be an overthinker. Welcome to the club. My name is Jill, and I'm also an overthinker. If you're like me, you probably know it's a problem. Maybe also like me, you haven't broken the bad habit yet. If this sounds a bit like you, know that you are not alone. I wish I had a magic wand to take away this all-too-common human trait of self-doubt and fear. Overthinking can take up so much of our time and energy if we allow it.

Since I still haven't found a magic wand for overthinking, instead, I will share a few tools in case it can help you.

Growth Tool

Stop The Thought Spiral

As a chronic overthinker, it is a constant and daily struggle to keep ourselves from spiraling on unhelpful thoughts. To ease that burden, try these three steps:

1. First, identify what you can control and what you can't.
2. Next, objectively identify what is true and let go of the inaccurate or unrealistic thoughts and feelings.
3. Then, counteract those unhelpful thoughts with an exercise in gratitude. Focus on what you can be grateful for at that moment, on that day, or in that week.

It's a start. Working to shift your mindset from the negative to something more positive and productive can do wonders. So much weight can be released from our burden of thoughts with these three steps. By creating positive thinking habits, in time, you can learn to stop your spiraling thoughts.

Growth Tool

Put Your Thoughts to Sleep

If you find yourself having trouble going to sleep or staying asleep because your thoughts keep you up, I've been there and it is no fun! Something to try is keeping a notepad and pen by your bed. If the endless to do list or worried thoughts start, simply write them down. Allow your brain to rest knowing those thoughts and responsibilities can wait until daylight. Write it and forget it, at least for several hours so you can sleep. We are more productive and effective if we are well rested. Sometimes a sleep aid helps too, practice a healthy evening routine to encourage good sleep and restful thoughts. Here are eight ideas to set a good routine:

1. Have a consistent sleep schedule. Wake up and go to bed at around the same time to train your brain and body.

2. Be physically active as regular movement and exercise helps you fall asleep and get better quality sleep.

3. Make sure you have an environment that encourages sleep: quiet, dark, cool, comfortable, minimal clutter, and no screens.

4. Create a relaxing bedtime routine: warm shower or bath, gentle stretching, meditation or listening to soothing music, reading a book, and avoiding electronics 30-60 minutes before bedtime.

5. Go to bed when you're tired. If you don't fall asleep within about 20 minutes get back up and do a relaxing activity until you're tired enough to go to bed.

6. Use alcohol in moderation as it can interfere with good sleep.

7. Cut down on caffeine and avoid having it late in the day.

8. Avoid napping or limit to no more than 30 minutes and not late in the afternoon.

Growth
Tool

Do a Body Scan

If you try to think away your stress and problems, you may actually be losing touch with how your body is holding onto stress. So, in moments when you catch your thoughts spiraling—PAUSE—and do a body scan. Start at your head or your toes and focus on each part of your body and how it feels. Release any tension. Be aware of your body's response. Be aware of your breathing.

The mind is powerful, and we can't bypass how our thoughts cause feelings, and in turn affects our body. If all else fails, I pull up my power song list and sing or dance my stress and anxiety out. Sending you loving and relaxed thoughts my fellow overthinking humans!

Dealing With Fear of Rejection/Fear of Failure

Trying new things or doing an activity you haven't done in a while can cause doubt and fear. If you are stepping into a new social situation, many thoughts may begin to race through your head. What if people reject me? What if I have nothing to talk to people about? What if I embarrass myself?

What if no one wants to be my friend? What if I offend someone? What if I ask and they say no?

What if...   What if...   What if...

I try to reframe that voice to say, "What would it hurt?" If you choose to put yourself out there, what would it hurt? No reason to jump to the worst-case scenario and talk yourself out of something that could be fun or even helpful. Try to remember the other people involved likely have these same fears playing in their heads. It's those darn bullies in our brain coming out to play. It's helpful to practice and use your tools to release the weight of these thoughts. If you are overwhelmed by your overthinking, I suggest you talk back with a more positive message. Remember, we will all get a no sometimes. Don't stop asking. We will all offend someone at some point or get offended. Don't stop communicating and remember to act with grace and compassion. We all run out of things to say sometimes. It's okay to let others fill the silence or to pause and know that sometimes silence is okay. We will all get embarrassed at some point. Try to find humor in it and take life less seriously. We can't be friends with everyone. It's okay to focus on quality rather than quantity of friendships.

Overthinking doesn't only impact social situations and personal relationships, it can hit hard in our careers too. Putting ourselves out there for new opportunities can be intimidating, scary even. At times we let this fear paralyze us to where we avoid change at all costs. If you are at an intersection of new and old or choosing your best path forward—I am cheering for you! If anxiety about big or even little career or life changes is creeping in, take a moment with me really quick, will you?

Growth
Tool

Manifest Positive Thinking

Take a moment to think of and envision the potential positive outcomes of the change or choice you are facing.

Breathe in confidence	Breathe in focus	Breathe in courage
Breathe out self-doubt	Breathe out distraction	Breathe out fear

If you too are an overthinker and human, and what-ifs and new situations cause you stress and anxiety, hang in there and keep using your toolbox!

The Lies Our Bullies Tell Us

At times our thoughts can get jumbled and it's hard to tell the truth from the lies. Some bullies are encouraged by outside sources. Whether you focus on thoughts you have of yourself, words you've heard others say to or about you, and even how others' actions make you think about yourself—learn which to listen to.

Growth
Tool

How to See Through the Lies

Start by writing down the words you hear from friends, family, and others in your life. Separately, write down what you say to yourself or think about yourself. Do they match? If not, this is a chance to reflect and assess. Identify where the bullies are living, identify the false and negative thoughts. This can also be a helpful exercise in finding toxic relationships whether with your own thoughts, or specific people in your life. Not sure what I mean? Here are a few examples of bullying thoughts, perhaps you've heard them or maybe you are the one thinking them (and I sure hope you are not saying these to others).

"If only you were..."
"You aren't enough..."
"You are too much..."
"If anyone really loved you..."
"Why can't you just..."
"Why aren't you..."
"Why can't you ever..."
"You're so sensitive, emotional, dramatic..."
"I was only kidding. You just can't take a joke..."
"You always..."
"You never..."

If you're thinking or feeling any of the above, take a moment to consider why you are giving these thoughts power. Are they true weaknesses you could work to improve, or are they a story in your head built by others? One way I worked through my bullies was getting more specific in my lists.

When considering the messages I heard from others, I broke it down further to who specifically I experienced this with. I considered whether these messages were ones I heard from most people or a select few. I took a moment to pause and try to look at these thoughts with an open mind instead of a defensive one. By pausing and looking at the bigger picture we can recognize if it may be a true weakness we can learn to improve and grow from. We can try to identify if it may be a thought imposed upon us by someone else's insecurity or fear. It's important to also admit we can all be victims of self-doubt spirals and misinterpreting the words or actions of others.

Growth
Tool

Don't Feed the Bullies

Sometimes these bullies come out to play when we are feeling weak or when we've neglected our self-care. Identify if there are certain times or situations that are triggering these thoughts. For me, I recognized some scenarios were creating a perfect storm and I was actually feeding into my negative thought patterns.

- Assuming bad intentions or judgment from others
- Not sleeping well
- Late at night when loneliness can be a factor (kind of like Gremlins, nothing good happens after midnight)
- Too much social media
- Comparing myself with others
- Being around people who are negative, critical, or judgmental
- Allowing the words and actions of others to impact my self-worth or self-love
- Indulging too much (for me it was food or alcohol)
- Avoiding conflict
- Not living truthfully
- Manipulation
- Feeling lost or out of control
- Poor communication
- When words or actions don't match intentions

Write Some of Your Triggers: _____

_____

_____

Give Those Bullies Some Back Talk

Now that I've hopefully opened your eyes to some of the ugly untruths, see if you can identify your patterns that tend to welcome those bullies in. Then, let's talk about how to pick ourselves back up once we've been pushed down. This is one situation where a little back talk is encouraged. Stand up for yourself and kick those hurtful thoughts to the curb. Don't start seeing yourself through your own self-critical thoughts. You determine your value and worth, no one else does! Once you see your worth and value yourself, the rest is a cakewalk. So, choose your words carefully, even the ones you don't say out loud. Take some steps to plan how you'll talk back the next time those bullies show up.

Make a Defense Plan

- Avoid the triggering habits, people, or situations as much as possible.
- For each trigger, come up with a plan of how you can realistically avoid or manage it.
- Make and keep a list of good thoughts.
- Repeat these good things as much as you need until the value of the message is felt and understood to be true.

Growth Tool

Remember Your Truth

Here are a few ideas to get you started.

"I am proud of myself."
"I choose what I become."
"I am likable and fun to be around."
"I am attractive."
"I am loved."
"I define my worth and I am worthy."
"I can do tough things."
"I work hard."
"I am strong."
"What I'm doing matters."
"I make a difference in the lives of people in my life."
"I am human and imperfect, and that is okay."

Write Your Own Good Thoughts! _____

_____

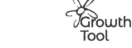

Growth Tool

Redefine Your Value and Worth

You and only you define your value and worth. Get specific and write out some comebacks for those bullies that keep showing up. Here are a few I use if you want to use, adapt, or add to them.

"I have value regardless of..."

My job
What I wear
Where I live
My productivity

My bank balance
The number on the scales

Write Your Own Comeback! _____

"I am good enough regardless of..."

What others think of me
Any mistakes I've made
My marital status
The behavior of my kids
My past
How I look
How many friends I have

Write Your Own Comeback! _____

Our thoughts hold great power. It's up to us to focus and prioritize the healthy thoughts, to choose the people, places, and things that bring us good energy. Let's step back from unhealthy habits or toxic relationships that keep letting these bullies in. May we all continue to work on stopping to be so fast to accuse and judge ourselves and others with our thoughts. Let's quit measuring ourselves by what we are or aren't accomplishing, or how we measure up to others. What we need to measure is what is in our hearts and how we treat others. We can control our intentions and actions. Once we start talking back to or ignoring those bullies in our brain, we can open our life to listening to the truth about ourselves and others. Why should we believe anything that opposes the truth we know in our hearts? Life is full of rejection, but this is one rejection we can control. Today and every day, be kind to your mind! Once we learn to play nice with ourselves, we will also play nicer with others. So, get out of your head already—exhale and move forward.

The Great Technology Disconnect

When interacting with others, how often are we on our phone when a person tries to engage with us about something, and we don't fully give that person our attention? If we can't break our focus, or if we respond with irritation or anger for having to transition our engagement, that is the problem. In that moment, our need to engage with our phone appears to be more important than the person trying to engage with us face to face. If we can't pull our eyes away long enough to fully look and listen to the human in our presence, and respond with attentiveness—what message are we sending them? Whether it's a family member, cashier, someone in the waiting room beside you, a food service worker, a neighbor, friend, or even your coffee barista—do they not deserve a moment of your attention? An acknowledgment of the person in your presence is all it takes. A moment to let that human feel seen, heard, and valued.

Now, with the technology humans juggle, there may be times when we need to respond to an important work email or any number of things that feel time-sensitive and important. If it is critical, it still doesn't take much time to simply look up and acknowledge the person you're with. If it is someone in your personal circle, it could be as simple as saying something like, "I hear you and I want to give you my full attention. Please give me two minutes to finish this message I am sending, and then I'd love to hear what you have to tell me." If it's someone in your public circle, it could be as simple as putting your phone down, looking the person in the eye, and sharing a quick exchange.

Again, if we respond with irritation, impatience, or anger for having to transition from a screen to a face in front of us—what are we teaching children who are watching the behavior we model? What is it doing to our relationships? I know this likely isn't a new thought, we've probably heard it and have been thinking about it. However, thoughts and words don't matter unless they are backed with action. I'm not saying to go back to a time of no cell phone or computer technology. Technology has brought about wonderful advancements and opportunities. Let's pause though and consider what slight changes we can make in our usage to bring back caring and respectful engagement.

Growth
Tool

Technology Cost/Benefit Exercise

Let's take a step back and look at this through a business mindset. If we look at the need for technology as being primarily about business; what are the costs and benefits of using our various devices? If we look from that vantage point, we can more easily see where we want to spend our time and energy. So, here's a little exercise I want you to try. Whether you do this as an individual or as a household is up to you. If you do not live alone, the most interesting method would be to have each person in the household do this and then compare your answers. If you are single, it's good to make time to reflect and take account of how you are spending your time.

- Take out a paper and first write down all the most used devices in your home.
- One by one, make a pros and cons list—an honest to goodness pros and cons list.
- Once you've done this, sit with it for a second and determine:
- What value does it bring to your life, on a scale of 0-10?
- What is its cost (not just monetary, but quality-of-life value too)?
  Now the purpose of this exercise is to recognize if there are things you can do to lessen the cost.
- Are the costs worth the benefit?
- Are there expectations or boundaries you can place on this to help bring more value and ease the costs you are experiencing?

I know we are all different and use technology in diverse ways. Technology has brought us entertainment and improved communication tools in our lives. But it's a matter of figuring out what are your true needs with technology and what aspects of it fall along the line of a want. Again, I'm not saying technology is the enemy, what I am saying is many have let it become the source of brokenness in our homes and relationships. If we know it is broken, why aren't we doing the work to fix it? Yes, I understand the fear of having to do the work to break habits. Unhealthy bad habits can be hard to break, but that doesn't mean we don't do the work to do what is right. Figure out what is right for your household and yourself. Find ways to unplug, reconnect, and get back to what matters. Create opportunities for sincere and authentic connection.

Online Engagement

I've been thinking a lot about communication and engagement (it's my business after all). We all engage with social media differently based on many factors in our lives and personalities. In modern life, we can't always be together in person. Surely you've considered how we've moved many of our connections with people to online spaces. However, have you shifted your thinking and actions to how you can better engage with people online? **Whether on social media or in person, people should act in ways that align with their character. Online platforms are not an excuse for poor behavior.** Sadly, we are seeing poor behavior more often with what may be perceived as a feeling of anonymity since people are separated by a screen. The way I see it, social media can be a helpful tool or a weapon, depending on whose hands it is in and how they choose to use it. So many blame the platform for a breakdown of many things when it is the people using it who are at fault.

So, how do you show up online? There are some people that share a lot and open conversations; they engage with people in kind and caring ways. There are others who simply scroll; they look and take it all in but are not engaging. They are not contributing to an online conversation or the groups and communities they have chosen to belong to. How are you showing up on these online platforms? If you are choosing to be on them, what are you there for? Are you there to make an impact? Are you there to connect with your community? Are you there for distraction? What are the things you are hoping to get out of it and how are you engaging in a way to achieve those goals?

The way I look at it, when we can't talk to each other in person, the way we engage with people online still represents ourselves. So, are you being authentic? Are you someone who when you walk down the street you would smile, give a friendly nod, or say hello? Are you doing that same thing online? If something engages or inspires you, are you pausing your scroll? Are you giving feedback? **By liking a post or commenting, it's the same as smiling at someone or engaging in friendly conversation.** If you want those conversations and deeper connections with the people you are choosing to have within those communities online; don't just scroll—pause—and engage. I challenge you to show up the way that you would in real life online.

Whatever you are choosing to show up for and spend time in, make sure you are using your time wisely. Make sure you are getting something out of it, but also make sure you are putting something back in. We can do better to connect, to continue conversations, to grow, and to support each other if we choose to stop our scroll and engage.

With online engagement, we also have the disadvantage of being able to hear a person's tone. We can't see their non-verbal communication cues. Read and interpret with so much grace. When we can't be face to face, it's important to remember those are real people on the other end of that screen. We don't know what struggle or challenge they may be facing within their home or outside their doors. We don't know what wounds they may be actively trying to heal. Work to acknowledge that the unkind or hurtful words we may receive often come from a place of hurt. Remember when you receive unkindness, it is more about the giver than the receiver. The way you respond to unkindness, whether online or in person, now that is all about you. It can be a great time for reflection and growth.

So, think for a moment—are you one that scrolls through, or do you stop and like or comment on posts? Do you find yourself getting swept up in arguments or reacting in negative ways you would not in person? Consider how that slight interaction may impact connection with others. Quit scrolling—pause and engage, in a positive and productive way! Choose to bring friendly and helpful interaction to our virtual communities. Assume the best in others and engage with good intentions. Remember how I said those we engage with online are part of our community as well? Don't hide behind a screen, use your words for good. Do your best to spread kindness, it's contagious.

Toxic Relationships and Bad Habits

When it comes to having a happy and healthy life, we must consider what things to add, remove, or adjust in our daily lives to help us feel our best. We must be self-aware enough to recognize what experiences, people, or things are adding or taking away from our good energy and overall wellness.

Recognition is just the beginning. Then we must lean into our courage and motivation to make a change and stick with it. Perhaps it's taking a big step and ending a toxic relationship, whether it be with a friend, family member, or colleague. Consider if there is a habit you have created that is working against you. Ending a relationship can be hard. It can feel like you're giving up. This is where I challenge you to see it differently. You are not giving up; you are standing up for yourself. You are not walking away; you are choosing to walk forward in a way that serves your life better. You deserve love, you deserve kindness, and you deserve respect. You deserve to protect your heart and the good energy that fuels your life.

Before I go on, a critical point:
Do not mistake toxic with abusive. Abuse is an extreme form of toxicity, and it should not be tolerated by anyone, for any reason, for any amount of time. If you or anyone you know is trapped in a physically, sexually, or emotionally abusive relationship, please take action. The National Domestic Violence Hotline is available for 24/7/365 guidance at 1-800-799-7233. Everyone deserves a healthy relationship.

Growth
Tool

Warning Signs of Toxic Relationships

Sometimes toxic relationships can build in subtle ways. These are some things you might start to notice:

- **Avoidance** – you avoid each other more and more or shut down instead of working through issues. You may find yourself trying to avoid conversations with the person or you'll bury your true thoughts and feelings and keep it to small talk to avoid a negative response.

- **Lost relationships** – you stop spending as much time with certain family or friends to avoid conflict. You may even feel like you've lost yourself.

- **Lack of support** – you feel unencouraged or unvalued, you don't celebrate each other's strengths and successes, only one person seems to be doing the work and trying.

- **Toxic communication** – conversations are filled with sarcasm, defensiveness, criticism, passive-aggressiveness, mocking, eye-rolling, belittling, scoffing, and hostility.

- **Lack of compromise** – unwillingness to admit fault, always wanting to be right, not being able to disagree in a respectful way and come to an understanding.

- **Nothing gets resolved** – too many conversations end in an argument and no resolution.

- **Resentment** – holding grudges, keeping a scorecard, everything is a competition, empty promises, bringing up past mistakes.

- **Constant stress** – constantly feeling on edge/walking on eggshells.

- **Persistent unhappiness** –you find yourself feeling sad, angry, anxious, or just hollow instead of joyful.

- **Change in mood/behavior** – you find yourself enjoying your time away from the person more than your time with them.

- **Envy** – you find yourself looking and comparing yourself to happy couples.

If the people in your life are not giving you what you need and deserve, it's time to make a change. There is a chance if you start seeing or feeling any of the signs listed above it may be a toxic season of your relationship and not necessarily a toxic end. Speaking from experience, my husband and I have been through some hard seasons that became toxic because one or both of us wasn't handling it well. Remember the earlier you put your hurt and concerns out in the open, in a productive way using respectful and empathetic communication skills, the sooner things have a chance to heal. Emotional and mental harm can be serious, and if you find yourself in a bad cycle, you'll have to decide if it's possible to work through the issue. Counseling, if both parties are willing, may be a great tool to help in that decision process. **As relationships go through transitions, we have to give up the idea that it's always 50/50 in effort, attention, or even intention. Instead, think of it as each person putting in 100% of what they can at that time.** We need to be realistic that relationships ebb and flow as life gets busy and everyone is at a different place in their wellness journey and ability to invest time in others. It takes both sides putting their best forward, acknowledging where weaknesses or pain points exist, and willingness to learn and grow.

So, choose your relationships carefully and ensure that if you are putting your time and energy into them, you are getting something you want out of them too. My advice is to never beg for a friendship or relationship with anyone. If they aren't matching your effort and adding to your glow—let them go. Your heart deserves better! You glow differently when you are surrounded by the right people, and it helps light your path. People in your life should be there to hold space for you and to listen. The right people won't want to change you or tell you who to be. Good people care to know you and all the wild pieces of your heart. They want to see you succeed and will be there to encourage you even when you fail. We are human, we are all a bit broken and beautiful. Surround yourself with the people who love you, broken pieces and all—they are your people!

It is important to remember not all toxic relationships are with people. Perhaps it's a bad habit. Life is all about balance and moderation to get to the healthiest and happiest version of ourselves, right? The reality of being a human is we'll have good times and some struggles too. In times of struggle, we may fall into coping mechanisms or unhealthy habits that do not serve us long term. We typically all make decisions at some point in life we are not proud of. We do not have to let those decisions define us! Drugs and alcohol tend to be a crutch or coping mechanism for some people that is rooted in deeper issues. I admit, in the months leading up to my mental health crisis, I leaned on alcohol at night when everyone in my house slept and I was up overthinking life. The situation was not helped by a worldwide pandemic, and I found myself more stressed and anxious without my regular social outlets. I fell into a habit of trying to numb my feelings and thoughts when they started to run wild at night. Instead of enjoying a beer to celebrate life's happy moments, it became a habit that made me feel sadder, more alone, and led to negative spirals of thinking.

I realized this trend and luckily was able to make changes to correct the habit. I still love good craft beer but choose to drink with good intentions and for happy reasons with family and friends—not by myself in times that are sad. This is still an area I struggle with at times. If I notice my consumption going up, I'll take a break and mix it up with some tasty non-alcoholic options. Luckily for me, a friend had already started a sober journey and shared all sorts of great recipes and tips through her new brand Decidedly Dry!*[6] If you are struggling with substances to avoid or distract from your feelings, chronic pain, or any other reason—please talk to someone. SAMHSA (Substance Abuse and Mental Health Services Administration) has a treatment line that may help, 1-877-SAMHSA-7. SAMHSA's mission is to reduce the impact of substance abuse and mental illness on America's communities. There are other ways to handle and cope with what is bothering you. You can still have wildly good times and not destroy your wellness. I am an advocate for good craft beer, but not at the expense of health, happiness, and lasting relationships. It's important to know what triggers you to feel genuinely happy just as much as it's important to know what triggers you to feel stressed, anxious, or sad.

Another toxic relationship I have made strides in but continue to work on is my relationship with social media. I know some of you will be able to relate to this. Again, in the evenings was when it hit me hardest. The mindless scrolling, the compulsive checking, the feelings of wanting to connect with people outside of my house all became a problem and at times made me more disconnected from my own family. I found myself creating habits of sharing too often, too much, or with the wrong people. It's a tricky balance at times. I still feel justified in my engagement and sharing. I know I have been successful in connecting people and resources within my local community. So, there are people who have directly benefited from the interaction in real life as well. I continued to say if what I was sharing helped even one person not feel alone, or helped one person to feel encouraged, then I had done something worthwhile in sharing. I believed I was helping people, and that brought me enjoyment. Social media is also a reasonable way for me to stay in touch with family and friends when we can't be together. Those pieces weren't so much the trouble. It became toxic when I began to crave certain interactions and engagement. It began to fill a bucket in my life that was not being filled elsewhere and it became more of an addiction. I felt seen, heard, valued, and appreciated. I realized I was leaning on this engagement at times as an excuse to escape my life and not work on what was missing or broken. I sought out more validation and attention and when I didn't get the interactions I had hoped for, it put me

---

[6] Resources included at end of book

into a negative spiral of self-doubt. Seeking so much validation through an online platform was destroying my wellness.

Growth
Tool

Make a Plan to Create Healthy Boundaries

I still have a way to go on getting out of the social media tailspin. At times, I still find myself compulsively checking things or spiraling into thoughts of self-doubt. I have been able to set some boundaries and utilize some tools to help though. Perhaps some of these may be a starting point for you:

- I have disconnected from people, pages, and groups that don't bring me good energy or tend to be timewasters.

- I have limited how many posts and stories I share to a lesser number.

- I limit my "friends" to only people who I have personal connections with in real life.

- I have worked to have more intentional engagement when I am logged in, with less and less mindless scrolling.

- During "family time," I put my phone away to avoid the distraction and allow me to focus on who and what matters in those moments.

- In the evenings I now often pick up a book, watch a show, or simply go to bed.

- I started counseling and have been learning ways to validate my sense of worth and value, regardless of outside sources or people.

- Instead of sharing all my thoughts and feelings on my Facebook feed, I began journaling.

The interesting thing with toxic habits is sometimes they can be masked in a good trait. Too much good can in fact at times be bad. If we're constantly doing good for others, we can end up neglecting ourselves. Whether we call this people-pleasing, being a fixer, toxic positivity, or whatever name you want to give it, this was an area I had to come to terms with when I was receiving treatment in the hospital. Amidst the hard, I was trying to find a silver lining to ensure some good came from that tough time. I was trying to see the good in people who were going through difficult moments. I wanted to offer grace knowing I too was not my best self at times. In my second week at the mental health hospital, after I had made some friends, because I thrive on connection with others, I had a bit of a wake-up call.

Although it was great to have a connection, I had to acknowledge everyone was working through their own challenges and trial and error with medication, just as I was. I had to remind myself to be mindful of red flags with other patients. I had to advocate for my own care and safety. There was one guy I had talked quite a bit with that at one point said he was having thoughts of raping me. It made me uncomfortable, but I wanted to give the benefit of the doubt. Maybe he was having trouble filtering his thoughts and he wouldn't follow through with what he said. Assuming the best in others like this can get me in trouble when it gets to a point where I don't grapple with the possible negative outcomes or realities of a situation. I ended up telling the staff and they had me sleep in a community room they could lock to ensure I stayed safe. At another point, I offered to switch rooms to offer support and be a roommate to a new patient that was admitted who had the same diagnosis as me. Soon after some heightened interactions, I realized she was in the early stages of harmful behavior. I had to back step from my offer to help her and recognize that may not be good for my own wellness and progress. These were just two examples of when I had to let go of the ideas that I could help or fix others to feel or be better. I had to put myself first and realize I was not there to help anyone else.

To achieve a good life, we often have a mountain to climb. A mountain range if you will. We carry an illusion that we'll find some amazing view at the top. Maybe some do, and for others, it may be the learning from the challenges on the way up that makes the way we see things differently by the time we reach the summit. I'd say the main goal is to not require a helicopter rescue, so we need to pace ourselves and surround ourselves with kind, compassionate, and loving people. We need to choose our actions with care, as actions become habits over time. We must be prepared for challenges and have supportive and fun-loving people in our lives. If you're going to climb a mountain you want to have the right people beside you every step of the way to make sure you are smiling and sharing some laughs as you work your way up! As you exert energy to continue your climb, you'll continue to discover new people who are great to walk beside on your journey if you leave yourself open to it.

Exhale and Move Forward

The journey to happiness doesn't happen in a giant leap but in many small steps. What are you stumbling on? There are times we are moving forward and then fall a few steps back. It's about figuring out what our next step is. Know and trust that each step can provide significant improvement in your life and the lives of those around you. With each little step forward, you are making an impact on your life and experience for the good. So, spend your time wisely, choose your actions with care, and continue your steps forward.

Growth
Tool

Create Your Plan for Personal Growth and Follow It!

Start small. If taking your next step feels daunting, think of it this way—if you had a magic wand, what three wishes would you make today? To be realistic (as you probably don't have a personal magic fairy) the wishes have a few restrictions:

- Each wish must be something you have the ability and control to change.
- One wish must benefit yourself.
- One wish must benefit your family.
- One wish must benefit someone outside your family.

Some people don't believe in wishes, and you're allowed to believe whatever works for you. I encourage you to think of wishes as your intentions. Each day we can make a wish, take the right steps, and choose the right actions to make them come true. We hold more power than we give ourselves credit for and hold our potential back because of fear or irrational beliefs about what we can do. Embrace your inner magic and move forward with your day! Wishes don't grant themselves; they take work.

The difference between a wish and a goal is a plan. Now how are you planning to make your wishes come true? If we want to find success, we need to cultivate the growth of our wishes as we would a garden.

Everything grows with love, consistent work, and intentional effort. As we plant our seeds of impact in our families, communities, and the world, we must do it with great care. To see it grow, we must continue doing the work to provide the right water and sunlight to ensure growth. We all have the choice and opportunity to bloom where we are planted. We can choose to see the struggle, but instead, I encourage you to see the opportunity for success, even in challenging times.

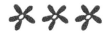

words to grow by

"What lies behind us and what lies before us are tiny matters compared to what lies within us."

Ralph Waldo Emerson

"You must not lose faith in humanity. Humanity is an ocean; if a few drops of the ocean are dirty, the ocean does not become dirty."

Mahatma Gandhi

"As you grow older, you will discover that you have two hands, one for helping yourself, the other for helping others."

Audrey Hepburn

"Be so busy improving yourself that you have no time to criticize others."

author unknown

"Seeds of faith are always within us; sometimes it takes a crisis to nourish and encourage their growth."

Susan L. Taylor

Chapter 6
Self-Care Is a Necessity, Not a Luxury

Everyone has a unique perspective on what will bring them happiness, whether it's their health, career, hobbies, relationships, or homes. What would you add to this list? For some, success can be perceived in all of those areas, yet feelings of true happiness often remain elusive. Regardless of everything we work to improve externally, the relationship we have with ourselves is at the heart of what makes our lives healthy, happy, and successful. The rest is the topping on the cake! We must quit hitting snooze and take action to focus our energy inwards to see a true difference! So much of our experience comes down to focus and energy. It is about progress, not perfection. It is about getting in touch with our focus and energy and recognizing how they can positively or negatively impact our lives. It is about taking care of ourselves first.

Your Life Is Like a House; Damage Can Come from Ignoring Regular Maintenance and Care.

Think of your life as a house. Let's say you walk into your house one day to find that the stairs have crumbled. Of course, you are shocked and overwhelmed as to how you'll get this fixed. Your mind goes straight to how much it's going to cost and how long it will take to find someone to fix the catastrophe. Why had no one told you there was a problem with the stairs? You stand there confused. You had lived here for years all by yourself and never had a problem with the stairs. Why have they crumbled now? In all the days, months, and years that you were going up and down those stairs, how had you missed noticing signs of a problem?

Situations like this usually start small and progress. In the past, you would only walk up the stairs to sleep in your room. At some point, perhaps you introduced a living partner or spouse—doubling the feet going up and down your stairs. Then, perhaps, your house became a home filled with a family and you'd go up the stairs carrying babies, laundry, and endless shuffling of things back to the rooms they belonged in. Maybe one day you added a home office. By then, you were going up and down the stairs to answer emails, do work, and address your other responsibilities. Thinking back, you begin to realize those stairs are supporting a lot more than when it was only you going up and down them to sleep.

Maybe you ask yourself, how long has this been a problem? You begin to remember that you noticed there were some squeaky parts in the stairs a while ago, but you didn't have time to fix them then. More recently, others in your house remember they noticed some loose areas where the stairs seemed weak. Again, life is busy, so everyone kept going up and down the stairs, ignoring the signs of damage, and not making time to do any maintenance or repair. Most recently it hit you, and you remember something looked off, almost as if someone had been taking out the screws holding the stairs together. You assumed someone else would surely notice and fix it, so you continued up and down.

What could've been a simple fix has become a bigger problem. Years ago, it may have taken a couple of hours to get the stairs supported and ready to use again. But now the damage is worse, the costs are higher, and the time it will take to fix them is immense. No one can use the stairs for weeks or months as you wait for the right repairs to be made.

In the end, it is our responsibility who we allow into our house and how we allow them to be a part of it. If there is a problem, we have to be aware of our part in it and how we can take positive action to improve it. When we noticed the squeaks, we should have investigated and addressed the issue. Small maintenance and care over time can help us avoid big problems from developing. With more strain on the structure, we have to check more often to make sure our house can hold up to that strain.

Lesson learned. In the future, if we notice there is a problem or something is starting to break or fall apart; don't ignore it, don't make it worse, and certainly don't assume someone else will fix it. If you notice something is not right—address it, talk about it, and take action. Unless we recognize and acknowledge what is wrong, we can't work to fix it. We don't always see what others see, so we must communicate.

Why Self Care Is Important

Like our homes, our lives need regular maintenance and care. We all need to pause from time to time to assess whether areas of our life need more support or are being overworked. All too often we hear work never rests, and some feel that to rest shows weakness, or to take time for self-care is selfish. Quiet those bullies in your brain, or those negative influences in your life. Choose to step away from the shoulds and self-imposed guilt or pressure and take a moment for self-care. Remember to listen to your body and give it what it needs so you can be your best self and show up well for others.

It can be easy to fall into thinking that rest is a waste of time when there are so many things to be done. I'm here to say work can wait, rest is a productive activity! Sleeping through life won't get you anywhere, but good energy can come from pausing long enough to care for yourself. Caring for yourself will in turn help you have a more effective tomorrow. Also, not all self-care is restful as we all recharge in different ways. Perhaps for you, it's running a marathon or climbing a mountain.

There is nothing wrong with taking a break from everything and concentrating on yourself. You are not responsible for fixing everything that's broken. You don't have to try to make everyone else happy. You are only responsible for your own wellness and happiness. Your peace of mind and health should be your priority. Everyone needs time for themselves to help them better focus and perform. So, make it happen!

This may sound daunting. Perhaps you don't know where to start. I say start small. Schedule it. Uninterrupted time takes planning. It's important to talk to those in your household so they know you'll be "off duty." Get their support for your self-care time. By taking time to recharge, it sets you up to be more productive in the time that comes after.

Growth Tool

Burnout Warning Signs

Burnout is a real thing—watch for the signs and take action to prevent it! Sometimes it's easier to listen and take care of the needs of our body than the needs of our mind. If you are feeling stressed, your mind and body are saying, "I need balance and signs of safety." Here are some signs of distress to be aware of that may be signaling you need to reprioritize your self-care.

- Amplified anxiety
- Change in appetite
- Detachment, apathy, loneliness
- Easily triggered
- Emotionally overwhelmed
- Exhaustion
- Feeling out of control
- Feeling resentful or unappreciated
- Frequent headaches
- Getting sick often
- Insomnia
- Little to no motivation
- More bad days than good
- Negative outlook
- Using food, drugs, or alcohol to cope
- Withdrawing from people

If you are noticing some of these warning signs you may need:

- A helpful mindset
- A safe environment
- Acceptance of self and others for who they are
- Advice, encouragement, community
- An uncluttered environment to unclutter the mind
- Culture, music, art
- Essential vitamins and minerals
- Fresh food, to be hydrated
- Helpful ways to cope with a challenge, solutions
- Influences of new and positive ideas
- Joy, love, release, purpose
- No unrealistic expectations
- Openness to learn and grow
- Real people connections, human touch
- Time to grow, learn, practice, love, and grieve
- To allow emotions to flow out
- To be in touch with nature, to touch, smell, sense, taste, and see

How to Make Time for Yourself

I'd like to challenge you (if you're not already doing it) to schedule "me time" in your day; even 30 minutes each day can make a big difference. When I went to the doctor after finding a bald spot (incidentally caused by stress), my doctor wrote a prescription on my take-home summary for "30 minutes of Jill time, daily." This time for ourselves can be a time for a creative brain break, physical activity, listening to music, or something else to distract from or soothe the responsibilities at hand temporarily. If you want to take it a step further, I say once a month, or even every other month, take a longer self-care break.

Again, scheduling self-care is important. For me, it is often outdoors and taking steps alongside friends. Other times it's a bubble bath and music or getting my hands dirty in the garden. We all have our "happy place." Get back in touch with the people, places, or things that make you happy and spend more time there. Your health depends on it! As the saying goes, **you can make time for your wellness now or you'll end up having to make time for your illness later.** There is no award for the one who is the most mentally, physically, and emotionally exhausted. To be healthy, happy, and successful, you need to show up as your best self, and being burnt out on life does not allow for that. As with anything else, starting small is the first step.

Growth Tool

Self-Care Through Trial and Error

Sometimes the biggest challenge is getting back in touch with what self-care looks or feels like for you. Here are a few ideas to give you a jump start —try some of these out and see what feels good for you:

- Snuggling up with a blanket and book
- Journaling
- Spending time by yourself, meditation
- Listening to music
- Going shopping
- Cleaning your space
- Cooking
- Massage
- Taking a warm bath
- Listening to a personal development podcast
- Painting, drawing, or some other creative outlet

- Going for a walk
- Sleeping in
- Spending time with a friend
- Lighting a candle or incense
- Treating yourself to a special drink
- Counseling, journaling
- Taking a break from negative people or influences
- Volunteering
- Taking a technology break

If none of these fit your version of self-care, experiment and figure out what is best for you. Find what brings you strength, comfort, calm, and encouragement, and then do more of that! When stress is high, the need to practice self-care is even more important. In those moments, double down on how you take care of yourself. Our roles in life change and shift, but the one constant is our relationship with ourselves. It should be our strongest relationship, yet often falls to the bottom of our list of priorities. It's easy to lose ourselves while being so focused on all the other roles we are trying to fill, and all the other people we are trying to take care of. Just like those airplane videos show us, you must put your oxygen mask on first. It will make you stronger and more prepared to handle whatever may be coming next. So, schedule it, plan it, and make it happen!

Since we're talking about scheduling, can we talk about counseling for a second? Although we are seeing some good movement in people being more open to counseling as a wellness tool, there is still quite a bit of stigma around it. Some think if a person needs counseling, they must be seriously broken or crazy. I started counseling, and if you are on the fence about seeking support, this is how I like to explain it: If someone kept passing out, they'd likely have to see a medical doctor to learn why and how to make it better. Perhaps the doctor would discover the person kept holding their breath too long or wasn't eating enough and would suggest corrective action for better health. The same goes for our thoughts and feelings. If we constantly bottle them up, they can negatively affect our health. If we don't feed our brain good things, it will suffer. The brain is a complicated and important part of our body and can require a specially trained professional to help. In my mind, counselors or therapists are a mix of a detective and a life coach for our mind and soul. Pretty cool if you ask me! It's like having your own personal cheering section in the game of life. They are there to help you find your best version of life and ways to work past the curveballs that life throws at you. Remember self-care is a journey, not a destination; we're bound to go over some speed bumps and face a few roadblocks and detours.

My Self Care Journey

I used to be the worst at making time for self-care. It would usually come about after my husband insisted that I take a break and a bubble bath, or he would encourage me to call a friend to meet up for a happy hour or walk. These were probably in the moments where he recognized my patience was running thin and I was not showing up as my best self. For me, it took an initiative I was selected to participate in to finally kick my butt into focusing on time for me. When it felt like a job, I was more likely to schedule it without that awful mom/wife guilt winning over.

It was 2017. I had a house full of boys aged 7, 6, and 3, as well as a consulting business which all together kept me busy and tired. My body and mind were screaming at me to find better health for myself, so I jumped into a new adventure of self-care. I had already stepped up to be involved as a Branch Ambassador for the Hike it Baby*[7] organization in my county the previous year which had been a terrific way to get myself out and active with my young kids. It was also a fantastic way to meet other nature-loving moms and families. I enjoyed nurturing my boys' love of the outdoors, but my focus was spent more on making sure they were happy, safe, fed, hydrated, respecting nature, and continuing to move one foot in front of the other. I was not prioritizing time for me to fully enjoy the trail.

So, when I heard Hike it Baby was going to launch the 10,000 Women Trail Project to get more girls and women on trails across North America, an initiative funded by REI's Force of Nature Grant, I was excited. The project offered an opportunity for women to encourage and bring other women and girls to get outside and spend more time in nature. I applied and was lucky enough to be chosen as one of the 100 Trailblazers across the United States selected to help get the project started and keep it going through the year.

In my role as a Trailblazer, I made it my goal to host ladies-only hikes and refocus on a little "me time." I continued this for the full year and once it was over, I realized I loved these fantastic women's days out! I loved this community of women. I could throw an adventure idea on the calendar, and I would almost always have someone jump on board. It wasn't just the hiking, it was the conversation, the relationships, and let's be honest, it was the typical brewpub stop after the hike too. If I am the one to plan an adventure day, guaranteed a stop with a delicious IPA is a must. It's like my dream date, and I got to invite my girlfriends to join me. Often it is while sharing a meal or on the carpool drives to and from the trailhead that we really get to know each other better.

After the initiative, and once my boys aged out of Hike it Baby, I chose to start a "Fresh Air Therapy" group. I knew I needed this once a month adventure day to continue in my life! The group name seemed fitting as the ladies who participate have mentioned how much they value and look

---

[7] Resources included at end of book

forward to these days. Something about it allows us to feel comfortable sharing what's on our heart and mind in this judgement free zone in nature. In pushing ourselves to try new things, go the extra mile, reach the higher elevation, and just be there to walk beside each other as we put ourselves first for a day, it offers such a healing experience and true soul refreshment. No matter the age, experience, or level of fitness—we leave no friend behind.

Now, years later, after adding friends and neighbors, we have nearly 80 ladies in the group. We've climbed mountains, swam under waterfalls, snowshoed in the dark, got lost a couple of times, cried together, laughed together, and shared some highs and lows of life together. Many didn't know each other before we started adventuring, yet a bond was made over a shared love of the outdoors. Sometimes it was only one other person, and sometimes it was ten. Through this group and the adventures, I built up my confidence. Confidence that I could do things on my own. I did a solo hike, nine miles, which I never would've been brave enough to do before and have done several since. I'll stop for lunch on my own and bring a book because there is also a strength that comes in having time alone and being comfortable in that space by yourself.

Big adventures aren't always possible, so during the pandemic, I also set up a weekly "Wellness Walk." It started with three little goals:
- Move my body
- Have real interaction with humans outside my house
- Invite all of my friends in case they needed it too

I used social media to set up these events and put myself out there. Was it a bit scary at first wondering if anyone would say yes? Absolutely! Anytime I put out an invite I worry about being rejected. Over time, and with the confidence I mentioned before, I am slowly getting better about stepping out on my own too. If no one shows, it's not personal and I still get out for my self-care time. These weekly walks ended up being something I, as well as a handful of friends, came to look forward to each week. A time that we could dedicate to our health and walk alongside each other to talk about whatever was weighing us down that week, or perhaps what things we could celebrate.

Looking back to when I started to prioritize time for myself, I can't help but feel thankful. Thankful I chose to seize the opportunity to enjoy life more. Grateful I had the opportunity to work on forming strong relationships and building community with others. Glad I had found ways to cope with stress that was healthier. As life has thrown me curveballs, handed me hardships, and tested me with big losses—this self-care journey became critical. By starting small, I could better handle the big stuff. I know I will not break down beyond repair. I know I can handle whatever comes my way and I appreciate that I have people to help support and walk beside me when I do fall. I am a people person, but I also love that through this we can each learn how to care for ourselves. That is the most beautiful of all. Self-love.

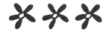

Chapter 7
Mental Health is Health

Self-care and mental health care are two strong pillars in what allows our lives to work well. I am passionate about normalizing the fact that mental health is a huge factor in our overall health, happiness, and success in life. Mental health has always been something close to my heart. Between my education in psychology, a background working with children and adults who struggled with various mental health conditions, and my family's personal experience with suicide due to mental health struggles; I know how important mental health and getting the right help and support is. Let's normalize therapy and medications that can help our minds stay healthy. Let's end the stigma. We need to be kind to our minds and encourage people to seek help before it's a crisis. Regular care and maintenance to keep our bodies in strong working order is important. **Our brains are an important part of our body and deserve no less care than other parts.**

Facing My Mental Health Reality

Let's rewind back to that day I crashed, both physically and mentally. The day my two-week nightmare began, a week after I drafted a book that I thought was going to change the world. The day I was admitted. I'll spare you all the scary details of those first few days in the hospital, but in short, I had an out of body experience. I felt like I was hit by a mental steam roller of possible diagnoses and top that with nearly every crime imaginable I thought I may have committed, or perhaps I was the victim of in this altered brain space. For a bit, I was sure I was dead, or that someone was trying to kill me. My mental health condition, in crisis mode, caused me to go into an extreme round of paranoid and fear-driven thoughts like nothing I'd ever been through in my life. I kept a journal at the time which helped me put together some of the details. Some of the experiences I know I will never forget for as long as I live, and others I wish I could. It was the most eye-opening experience of what those with mental health conditions go through. It was dehumanizing and the hardest thing I've ever gone through in my life.

It felt like a year of my life away from my family, friends, community, and anyone or anything I recognized. I survived those difficult days by trying to focus on simple things that made me feel some level of contentment each day. I needed to connect with things I enjoyed or that made me feel any ounce of normalcy. I listened to music I liked. I tried to find feel-good shows I was familiar with, *The Bee Movie* being one. My family was able to drop off a few items for me, so I had adult coloring books, word finds, dot to dots, magazines, and books with faith-filled words to help me distract and focus my mind away from where I was. I realized my brain was trying to associate the people at the hospital with any quality that reminded me of people I cared for and who cared for me in real life. Whether it was that black hoodie they wore, their facial hair or eyes, or perhaps the way they spoke to me that reminded me of someone else. I reached for anything similar that made me feel less afraid in an unrecognizable environment. I began to organize my paperwork and take notes on things that could be improved or made more effective in the running of the hospital to feel like I was being helpful or productive with my time there. I organized daily walks with other patients in the halls where I stayed to help encourage physical and emotional wellness as we would talk as we walked. It helped bring a sense of connection and community with those who were willing to step along with me.

I found ways, even in the hardest of times, to incorporate small bits of the types of self-care I had practiced at home. The habits I formed became critical during the two weeks I spent in the mental health hospital trying to find myself again. I became so thankful I had explored this journey of self-care. In an extremely basic triage sort of way, it helped. That is the wonderful thing about scheduling self-care and making it happen. By making it happen you are forming good habits, you are practicing good coping mechanisms for times when life gets hard and you need something to fall back on. It helps you to get back up when you fall. It allows you to pick up the pieces.

Mental Health and Self Care Journey Continues

Hopefully, these glimpses into my journey help you feel safe in sharing your story. May you feel better in knowing it's okay to talk about mental health, it's okay to seek help, and to understand it isn't a once-and-done experience. It's so important to check in with ourselves. As I said before, self-care is a journey, not a destination. Recently, I started to feel myself fading into that shadow of myself a bit, feeling less motivated, and just going along with what others wanted or needed from me. The year following my diagnosis was a hard season. My dad was diagnosed with brain cancer and passed away very suddenly. I lost eighty percent of my client base as well as a close friendship. The losses didn't stop there. My husband lost his job and then my uncle/godfather passed away after suffering with ALS (amyotrophic lateral sclerosis). Oh yeah, and in the mix of all that I got shingles (a stress-related winner), my husband got Covid, and then I got vertigo. At least my hair was growing back! These losses and hardships all happened over six months, right through the holiday season and through my milestone birthday of turning forty. Not much to celebrate at that time. I hadn't been able to have my regular counseling sessions as my counselor moved and I had been reassigned. So, with so many things piling on, I felt defeated. I did not feel emotionally and mentally strong. I recognized I was neglecting my healthy routines and habits and as a result I needed a pick me up!

So, one night when the family chose to stay home, I went on my own to listen to music down the road. I brought a book figuring I'd sit by myself, but after showing up, I saw there was an open firepit and just one person standing by it. I figured, why not join them? We talked about things other than our kids, and eventually, a few other guys came to stand around the fire and the conversation continued to flow. None of us knew each other, but it was enjoyable to be there together sharing a beer and talking about our jobs, hobbies, the beer industry, and a variety of topics—none of them mom-related.

As a parent, so often our conversations revolve around our kids. It can feel intimidating to remember how to have conversations with other adults; conversations that involve topics other than parenthood. We so easily forget other humans may find us interesting, and we can even forget what we are interested in. Funny how random little things can boost our confidence. I may have grinned on the way home that night, and again the next day. Proof I still got it, I can keep up with an adult conversation, and even be interesting! It's good to be reminded on occasion that we are individuals in all our unique and interesting ways. It's good to give ourselves permission to do things we enjoy on occasion, even if others don't choose to join. That night I was just Jill for a couple of hours, and I liked being with me again.

Practicing solitude is so important. If you can practice doing things and experiencing things by yourself while it is your choice to do so, it can build strength and self-awareness. It can build a sense of peace in learning that you can in fact enjoy doing things solo. If you always rely on others to make meaningful experiences, a time will come when you have no choice but to do something by yourself. If you wait, those moments or experiences of being alone may feel overwhelming, scary, or sad. If you have built up that practice of enjoying and finding peace in solitude, perhaps you won't have the pain of ripping off the band-aid when it is not your choice. Life is meant to be shared, so don't take this as instruction to abandon relationships and experiences with others. Nothing at all like that. Instead, embrace those small moments to be with and love yourself. Some day your future self may thank you for it.

Life gets busy, life can be hard, and life can throw things at us we are not sure how to receive or handle. I have had to remind myself to continue to work on prioritizing my wellness. Building mechanisms for self-care and support are critical to continue to move through whatever life brings. May you embrace whatever part of the journey you are on—you got this!

GROW THROUGH WHAT YOU GO THROUGH

Be Kind to Your Mind

Our emotional health can range from thriving to struggling. No matter what you're experiencing, there are ways to take action to support yourself and those around you. I had to come to terms with the fact I'll be on medication for the rest of my life to stay healthy. Luckily, the doctors found the genetic connection and the one diagnosis that fit my symptoms, Bipolar 1. The doctors got me on wonderful medicines to help wake me up from the nightmarish (although dreamy at times) reality I had been living. It was a mental health awakening, and no different than if I had a heart condition or diabetes that needed medication to regulate. It doesn't change who I am or what I can do! Like most things with our bodies, nothing fits into a perfectly prescribed mold. I have been nervous about sharing my specific diagnosis. Too often, the worst-case scenario or negative aspects of mental health experiences become the focus. I refuse to let the assumptions or judgments of others tell me how I am supposed to experience this as everyone is different. I am not naive to the condition I have. I want to share the good and the hope.

I share this part of my story because it's not something I should be ashamed of or hide. There is such a stigma around it, and people aren't as comfortable talking about it because there is still so much judgment to fear from others. Well, this is my step forward in saying don't hide from the truth. As I write this, I am pushing back against the stigma and all the preconceived judgments people hold about people who have a mental health diagnosis. I am here to say I appreciate and celebrate my brain for all its perfectly imperfect parts. I've been told many things about it over the years, but I know it is my strongest and most beautiful body part. Embrace all your parts, they make you who you are, and you are beautiful!

There should be no fear or shame around mental health and people should feel safe talking about it. If you or someone you know is living with a mental health condition, consider how you think of it. Be aware of how you feel and talk about it. I listened to a wonderful podcast recently called "Anxiety: Is It Just Love Holding Its Breath," which is part of the We Can Do Hard Things podcast series with Glennon Doyle.*[8] I strongly encourage you to follow this

---

[8] Resources included at end of book

series, it's great! Anxiety is just one of many mental health conditions. This podcast beautifully explains how we can choose to see anxiety as a feeling of intense love instead of worry or fear. Reframing how we see and talk about mental illness and the warriors who live with it matters. Instead of, how do I deal with this, think what gifts has this brought to my life. Instead of loving someone despite of their mental health, love them because of it.

Initially, when I learned I had a mental health condition, it was the most terrifying few weeks of my life. But luckily, I received help to get my brain and body healthy again. It was nerve-wracking to share this new part of my life. Thankfully, no personal electronic devices were allowed at the hospital as there were some great bloopers reels from those first few days when I was not myself. The only visual evidence from those days exists in my memory. Some memories I cringe about while others I can luckily laugh about. Humor can help get us through tough times, so I tried to find the humor as soon as I could. Those first few days (and a couple of weeks leading up) until I was diagnosed, the doctors found the right medicines, and my body adjusted out of crisis mode, there were some doozies. I guarantee some apologies were made for those early days. Part of the reason I share this writing and my story is to give hope. Hope that we can change the conversation around mental health. Change people's thinking that a diagnosis defines us. It doesn't. That needs to change! **People with mental health conditions don't have a life sentence, they have a life of opportunity. The opportunity to see the beauty in what their brain and life is capable of succeeding with.**

Our brains are all beautiful and our deep feelings just add to the experience and magic of life. That spirit and fire light life up, so don't feel you need to hide it away. Choose to be yourself and love others for all they are. I choose to embrace all of myself; the silly, imperfect, fun, different, happy, quirky are all part of my recipe. It's my real and authentic self. So, I encourage you to be you because life is too short to care about how others see you! Just be yourself—everyone else is already taken.

Chapter 8
The Keys to Success

With each new year, month, day, or hour that passes in our life we have a choice. Will you choose to go through life on autopilot and fade into the background of your life, or will you make the choice to stand out? Don't be afraid to show your true colors and chase your dreams. To live the version of life that makes you succeed and smile, you need to be willing to grow and work towards it. Are you settling for less because it seems easier? Are you stepping back from opportunities for fear of failing? Step away from that fear and be confident in the fact you get what you work for in life. I will be cheering for you to reach that next step toward your goals. Don't give up, especially on days you feel stuck!

The way I see it, the key to success is twofold: first, you must observe and understand the obstacles and opportunities occurring in the circumstances around you. Second, you must be able to see how your choices can have a positive impact on these circumstances. Your strength shows in how you listen, seek to understand, and empathetically respond in challenging situations. Observe and learn. Take the opportunity to pause and respond in productive ways, instead of simply reacting. This strength and confidence will lead naturally to sound decisions and effective actions that may be better received by others, and success and growth will follow. Leaning on self-awareness and compassion provides the right power to lead you to make good choices for the outcomes you desire. The key to success is strength and not the kind that overpowers others, rather the kind that looks to lift all to greater heights and leaves no one feeling stuck.

Growth
Tool

Redefine Strength

How do you define strength? What makes a person strong, a family strong, a business strong, and what makes a community strong? I believe the key to the success of the latter three is dependent on the strength of the first. It's a trickle-up effect, so to speak. For any community, business, or family to be strong and successful, it depends on the strength of the individuals and the leaders within it to be the foundation. Over time, my definition of strength has changed.

- Strength is not a person who has no weaknesses, but rather a person who acknowledges their weakness and continuously works to learn and improve.

- Strength is not a person who wins every race, instead it is a person who strives to do better in each race they run.

- Strength is not someone who never cries, but instead someone who experiences all their emotions, can identify then, and knows how to work through them.

- Strength is not someone who never falls, it is instead the person who gets back up every time they fall.

- Strength is not someone who is perfect, but it is someone who acknowledges they are human and takes accountability when they make mistakes.

- Strength is not someone who wins every debate, but rather someone who seeks to clarify and understand knowing most issues are not black and white.

What is strength through your eyes? What do you see as a key to success?

Engage With Kindness

Enough terrible things are spreading in our world, why not choose to share and spread the good! If you choose to bring a little spark of joy to each part of your day and live colorfully—it just might be contagious, and you never know whose day it might brighten.

Share a smile	Spread joy
Share your time	Spread hope
Share encouragement	Spread kindness
Share your resources	

Consider if your perspective may help others through what is challenging them in their day, or if what you are sharing adds to their challenges. Kind engagement doesn't have to be some big gesture. It's time we realign our lens to focus on the right things.

Kindness In Action

Showing kindness to others can be as simple as remembering:

- A handshake, a smile, and a kind word can go a long way in making someone's day good.
- Showing respect when we leave someone's presence.
- A simple goodbye, have a nice day, or it was so good to see you as you leave lets someone know you care.
- Making eye contact when we speak with one another.
- Speaking truthfully, with kindness, and good intentions.
- Opening a door for a stranger.
- Lending a helping hand to anyone in need when we are able.
- Respecting our elders.
- Knowing instant gratification isn't life.
- Remembering patience is a virtue, and to practice it.
- Appreciating if you want something in life you need to work for it.

These are simple ways to let another person know you value and respect your time with them. Our time with others has value and we need to get back to showing value with both our words and actions and choosing to engage wisely.

If You Cannot Offer Empathy, Offer Kindness Instead

Showing kindness to others means loaning your strength instead of reminding them of their weakness. We all cope with the rollercoaster of life differently based on our personalities, home environments, and life situations. We may not always understand what is causing the actions or communication we receive from others. Everyone is working through struggles each day. Our goal can be to open up the conversations and break down the stigma around sharing with others, by responding with kindness. We can make it okay to share both struggles and successes with others, without fear of judgment, shame, or pity. With each interaction we have, we can strive to understand or clarify what we don't understand. We don't need to return unkindness with unkindness. Our chosen words can either bring us together or separate us from each other. If we choose to communicate in ways that involve defensiveness, stereotypes, fears, and biases, it will break our connection with others. Instead, we need to communicate with empathy, understanding, kindness, and compassion. There is so much we don't see in others that affect our interactions and how we experience life. Respecting there is more to each human than what we see or at first hear can encourage us to approach our interactions with a bit more grace toward others as well. We each have a unique makeup that includes things like:

Single – Married – Divorced – Widowed – Parent – Grandparent – Friend
Neighbor – Republican – Democrat – Liberal – Conservative – Working –
Retired - Unemployed – In Transition – Blue Collar – White Collar –
Terminal Illness - Mental Health Challenge – Physical Disability – Optimist –
Pessimist – Introvert - Extrovert – Fixed Mindset – Growth Mindset

There is a rainbow of perspectives and views, and all bring their own colorful light to our world. When it comes to what we believe, we hold a variety of ideals based on our own personal interpretations. So, before you engage with someone assuming one of you is wrong and one of you is right, consider it may simply be a different perspective. You can think in ways that are considered old-fashioned, modern, liberal, conservative, or simply a dreamer beating to your own drum not thinking inside any of those boxes. Whether prayer, positive vibes, good energy, or whatever enriches you to the core is at the base of your beliefs—you do you! At the end of the day, we have to understand that variety is good. Learning to understand and learn from other viewpoints is what enriches society. I'm not saying we will agree on every issue, but let's work harder to disagree with respect and understanding. Let others believe what they want if it's not hurting you or anyone else for them to do so. Lead with kindness.

The Power of a Smile

In the wise words of Mother Theresa, "*We shall never know all the good that a simple smile can do.*" Have you ever noticed you can spot a kind person from across the room? You can see it in their eyes, you can hear it in their voice, and you can recognize it in their willingness to genuinely engage in a positive way with whoever is near them. Odds are you'll see them smiling or hear them laughing as they engage with others. Simple things, right? So, let me tell you a short(ish) story about a simple moment of kindness that helped me through a moment of discomfort and fear. One story I know is repeated throughout the world, but this little one is mine.

I had gone into the hospital one day for bloodwork and as I was sitting in the waiting room, I took out my phone for distraction to try to calm my nerves. I am terrified of needles. Just then, an older woman sat down nearby and in the kindest voice started a conversation with me. So, of course, I put down my phone, smiled, and gave her my full attention because that's how you show someone respect. By giving someone your eye contact and full attention, you are showing them they matter, what they have to say matters. I can't remember exactly how she started the conversation, but it could have been something as simple as the weather, complimenting something I was wearing, or sharing she had a challenging time hearing when they called her name when waiting at the doctor's office. We engaged in the simplest and most wonderful conversation. At one point an older gentleman with a cane came in and sat by us as well and joined in for a few words.

In that short little conversation, we talked about the values of a positive attitude, the value of patience, and trusting the process. We acknowledged how sometimes things are out of our control, and we can't control the timing, so we just have to go with the flow and know in the end, everything will turn out the way it's supposed to be. We talked about how life can be full of distractions and there are things around us we can't explain and don't have the answers to. How it's important to know when there are things that are not in our control, we have to trust the people in charge of it are doing their best to get it done right. Some things are not for us to question. We also realized we were probably related once we started sharing the last names of our relatives, the gentleman even recognized my grandma's maiden name as she grew up just a stone's throw from where we were.

This condensed version of the story goes to show we live in a small world and are connected in so many wonderful ways if we just pause, engage, and take time to ask the right questions. Sharing is caring and gosh I loved sharing these moments of smiles and laughs with Betty. I was so busy chatting I didn't hear them call my name, luckily, she was listening and let me know. I wish she knew how much that interaction made my day and surely one of the reasons why I didn't cry. I may never see her again, but this was a story worth sharing in hopes it inspires you to look at your interactions differently. Don't let the distractions of modern life keep you from engaging in these types of kind interactions with the humans around you in your daily life. Find ways to engage and share a smile!

Make Your Work Matter

If we are spending so many hours of our day working, shouldn't it matter what we're working on and who we're working with? Let's look at this from the bird's eye view—when I say work, I mean your life's work. I know that is a big picture view, but at the end of each day isn't that what truly matters? The big picture?

As you move into each new day remember to work on, or work toward, discovering what the passion and purpose are behind what drives you and work on that. Fill your day with that and spend your time wisely. Spend your time and energy doing what truly matters in the pursuit of success. Not just in your professional life, that's just one small box to check in this big picture of life. Wealth comes not through money alone, but in the richness of our relationships, experiences, and contributions to this larger puzzle we are each a piece of. Lead your life with passion and purpose, with an open mind and an open heart, and I believe at the end of the day you will find all the success in life you dream of. Time to think and live outside the box, think from the heart and it will lead you to extraordinary places!

I realize habits are hard to break. I continue to work on them myself. I've been a night owl for the last 12 years as I worked to juggle work and family once choosing to stay home to raise my babies and start my own business. I had this dream of having it all, work and family. Well, I'd been burning the candle at both ends, and it recently hit me like a laundry basket to the head that there may be—no—that there is another way. So in my darkest times, I decided why not start to do the arduous work to change what's not working in ways that serve the life I want? I mean truly, why am I spinning my wheels working so hard if I'm moving toward the wrong goals and in the wrong direction.

Backpedal with me for a second. The way I see it, we're all working so hard in these little boxes of life we are living in. Working in hopes of contributing to and achieving all of life's successes. How are you measuring success though? Wait, stop there! Think for a second about if perhaps, just maybe, the true success you need to be working harder for isn't inside that box you're sitting in.

So many sayings in life keep running through my head and this one rings true: Do what you love and love what you do. We hear this all the time, but do we do it? We feel like it's this impossible dream, unattainable, and only exists for the lucky few. I don't really believe in luck so maybe that's the difference. I don't believe that good things come to those who wait, I believe if you want good things you need to go out and find those opportunities. Opportunities in life don't come to us by chance, more often they come to us because of the choices we have made in life that put us in the right place, time, and mindset to be open to the possibilities that cross our path.

Life is full of doors ready to be opened if we simply go out and look for them. Don't walk past assuming it isn't the right door, that you haven't been invited, or the people on the other side of that door won't be happy to see you. Believe in yourself, have confidence, and sometimes in life it's okay to be a party crasher and boldly walk through that door. What will it hurt? Sure, there are times it's a bathroom door and that can feel embarrassing and you quickly backstep once you realize that was not your door of opportunity. Does that mean you quit opening doors, you quit being curious, you quit looking for the next opportunity? I hope not! Not all doors are meant for us, but we can't stop opening them and looking for the possibilities. You'll know when you've found the right one and I am so excited for you to see where it leads you! If I'm a stranger and am feeling giddy with excitement to see you succeed, I guarantee those in your corner of the world will be as well. Remember all those words about celebrating others, I believe it with all my heart!

I feel fortunate with the work I've done. I have found fulfillment in being a resource to people. I have helped make parts of life less stressful, or easier, for those I work with or for. In many ways, I became a fixer, a communication specialist, and a behind-the-scenes detail master. It's not like I sit staring at spreadsheets and data and feel excited. But I am happy that through sometimes repetitive tasks and detailed work I can find ways to help processes and systems work more smoothly or efficiently. It isn't always the actual tasks of the work that bring me fulfillment. When I deal with disgruntled customers or handle bad reviews online for my clients, I am not glad to face conflict. I am, however, thankful for my communication skills. I am often able to deescalate disgruntled customers with respect and empathy. I am often able to find the right words to respond in a way that is calm and helps people feel understood. It is the validation of knowing my customer or client trusts me with something they feel is especially important in their business.

Sometimes it's adjusting our perspective as not many get a perfect job they love every part of. But we need to **ensure our job, the work we do, and the business(es) we work for align with our vision of how we want to make an impact**. If we can find that, we find more fulfillment in what we do for so many hours of our day. For most of us, we're going by the idea we work to live, not live to work. Working isn't optional as there are bills to pay, but I feel it's important to ensure you are not miserable in your job as it is often a big part of our life and can be a big part of our identity. Yes, there will be times we persevere our way through a job because it pays so good it allows us to make an impact in other ways aside from the job. That is a slippery slope though as money can't buy happiness. Too often the stress, disappointment, overwhelm, resentment, or other feelings you may be picking up in your job spill over to your personal life. No job is worth destroying your quality of life, regardless of how big the paycheck is.

Being a Champion Is Your Choice

We each have a CHOICE as to how we spend our days. This choice impacts whether we will be a CHAMPION of the days ahead. What choices will you make in how and where you spend your time? Good choices are made with:

C ourage
H umility
O ptimism
I ntegrity
C onfidence
E nergy

What are things that can set you up well to be a champion of the days ahead?

C reativity
H ealthy Choices
A ltruism
M otivation
P erseverance
I nitiative
O pen Mindedness
N oble Character

Every person will experience life uniquely. Make a plan of how to make yours a success. What actions and steps do you need to take to get your life where you want it to be? Life is about more than looking sharp, it is about the work you produce. Be sure you are working to stand out in the right ways.

Harms of Hustle Culture

One day, I stopped for coffee and got one of those cups that has motivational words on it. I always enjoy seeing what inspiration I can glean from the words and messages I see throughout my day. So, I looked at the cup and here's what it said: "Get up early, Stay up late—Change the World". Yikes! That didn't inspire me and instead made me feel tired and like I couldn't possibly measure up to that suggestion. So, I chose to modify the message slightly: "Get up ~~early.~~ Stay up ~~late.~~ Change your life ~~the World~~."

Today's hustle culture can be harmful to our health and well-being. It can make us feel defeated before we even begin. Hustle culture is the unreal ideal that we need to burn the candle at both ends in order to be successful. An expectation that we are available and should respond to work at all times, even outside regular business hours. What I see as hustle culture being harmful is that there are often expectations that revolve around wants (not needs) that impose an unwarranted pressure that we feel we must fill. A giant expectation of success that most cannot reach. To change that culture, we must choose not to hustle to impress, to compare, to show we are worthy, to show we are enough, and to meet that unrealistic ideal that society places on humans in modern life.

There is a difference between hustle culture and hustling to survive. No one was built to carry the weight of the world, so let yourself set that load down. There are however times that we have to hustle to meet the needs in our life (not the wants). We must do whatever it takes. We have to work our tails off to make ends meet. Our lives can't always wait. We can't always sit back and take a break. There are bills to pay, insurance to find, medicines to fill, groceries to buy, true obligations that must be met. So sometimes we have to exhaust ourselves to meet the goal—the goal that can't wait. That's not the hustle I am talking about.

As for the rest—take a breath, take good care of yourself, and decide what goals and tasks truly matter in your life. Today you don't have to stay up late or get up early; you do not have to change the world. Perhaps today (and every day) it's enough if you get up, stay up, and do the work to change your life.

Celebrate Others

Has society become so focused on personal success that we forget to celebrate the success of others? Someone else's success is not a direct reflection of yours, so why not celebrate alongside them? Consider if you're running a race and made a personal record that day. That is worth celebrating, right? Perhaps you didn't come in first in the race that day, but you came in first in your race. When you pass the finish line, congratulate the person who did come in first, as it may have been their success for the day. Also, celebrate yours. Wherever we are in this race there will be people behind us and people in front of us, and it's best to focus our energy on where we are in that moment.

What matters is being able to stop and realize wherever we are in our race to the finish line, we can still cheer on those around us. Quit comparing and doubting yourself. Instead put energy toward seeing the good in others, celebrating them, and not letting that become a measurement of your own success or potential. We should feel joy in seeing one another succeed or having a good moment.

When it comes to business, I have to say I am most impressed by those that treat their competition well. Yes, we all want to earn the business, and being gracious when it doesn't land in our court is important as well. Being able to speak kindly of those that may provide the same service or product reflects well on you and helps to build relationships. We all have times when we need to refer out, or perhaps even partner with those in our industry. Best to play nice and then everyone can rise.

Keep Faith in Your Future

We all know the best things in life take time to grow. Your time will come! We plant many seeds, some grow, some die. In life, everything eventually dies, and the goal is to bloom into our full potential before we do. In blooming and sharing our growth, we can pass along our seeds to enrich future growth. We are all on our own journey of growth. It's a beautiful journey full of rainy and sunny days. Trust you can grow through a storm. Keep reaching for the sun and your rainbow will come when you open yourself to seeing it. If you find your secret to happiness, seek to help others find the path to theirs. By helping each other to see and be good, I truly feel our world will be a better place to live. Just like the best times of the good old days, time can be good again. Of course, with some improvements and advancements as that is the way it's supposed to be, constantly evolving, and changing. When we know better, we can choose to be and do better. You can do anything you put your mind to that you believe in your heart.

Life Is Tough, But So Are You

It may be true that life isn't easy. I don't think it ever really has been, there has always been stress in life. That doesn't however mean we back down from the tough things and just take the easy road. Through every struggle, hardship, or challenge, we learn and grow. As we continue to strive for advances in technology and business may we not lose touch with the heart of humanity. What good are all of the advancements if as people we are breaking what truly matters in the process? Consider if by focusing on the wrong things we are hurting what matters most. I think we see the writing on the wall, we see the damage done and the truth of what will come if we continue on the path we're on.

I also believe once we see the truth, we can work to change it. It is up to each of us to turn back the pages of this modern life story we are telling ourselves and realize it needs to be written better. We need to be more thoughtful of what we want to fill our lives with, what we want to prioritize in our homes, and what we want to feel.

Sure, this may seem overwhelming, it may seem hopeless at times to think any of us can possibly do anything to impact that kind of change. The truth is, we have so much power! We can do tough things. We can do remarkable things. We can make change happen. All it takes is you! It takes you dedicating your heart and mind to good. It takes you taking that first right step toward change. I genuinely believe all profound changes start with one idea, one good idea that is shared, encouraged and spreads. So why not spread the good instead of the bad? We keep saying the struggle is real, and it is, it absolutely is. The struggle is real because we choose to let it be. Why not instead of struggling, choose to focus on making our experiences a success? It all comes down to our choices. We make choices every day that all add up to the puzzle of life we are creating. You already know inside you the pieces you are forcing to fit that really don't compliment that picture you want to see. Why not instead focus your actions on the pieces you feel compliment the picture you want to see?

We're told to not focus on the past and to look toward the future. I think in forgetting to remember our past and what was great about it, with the focus to just charge forward, we lose sight of what we were already doing well. Do you know the saying if it ain't broke don't fix it? Well, my worry is in the process of advancement we ended up breaking what was working. We've broken our families, we've broken our communities, we've broken our communication, and if we don't change, we will break humanity. We can do better, we need to do better, and the time to do that is now. We cannot back down from the work we know we need to do for fear we'll fail. We are already failing. We have fallen so far from what we were put on Earth to do, and it is time to pick ourselves up and try again. We can no longer put off for tomorrow what we can do today.

Life Happens in Seasons

We all know life is a roller coaster of seasons and change. Whether you choose to be single, married, divorced, have kids, or no kids—every version has its own cycle. Life is all about moving forward, not back and trying to enjoy the ride through all the ups and downs. There are so many lows that affect us all. Those lows are what people tend to have a tough time talking about. I hope that will change, and if you are facing a dark time, I want you to know you are not alone. The people in your life have come there for a reason. You may not know it now, but if you open yourself to those around you, you will be supported in every way to get through uncertain or challenging times. If you open yourself to engaging and building community, over time, you will realize you have an ocean of support to help you through each wave and low point of life. We may not always be connected to the right people at the right time to help us through dark times. Sometimes the timing just doesn't work out. Those times are when you grow in your own strength. Know whatever you go through, you were built to handle it. You were built to withstand the storms that come your way.

I hope a few of these words help you to move to your next happy season. Remember to seek support and community through challenging times. Whatever you are experiencing, there is someone that has been through something similar, and in sharing your story you can walk through that time together and help one another.

Life Is Short – Live for Today

I continue to work my way through a journey of personal growth. As I reflect on this past year, instead of focusing on the struggle, I celebrate the success. It was a year that my hair fell out and thankfully grew back. A year where I thought I was dying and ended up having a mental health crisis that could be treated with medication. A year where I was in a terrible car accident and miraculously came out unharmed. A year where my dad unexpectedly got diagnosed with an aggressive form of brain cancer and died just 22 days later at the age of 65, and I was fortunate to be able to be with him and help care for him on so many of those final days. A year with so much unexpected loss, change, and uncertainty that I managed to stay afloat through and even thrive. It was a year that I, for so many reasons, came to terms more emotionally with the complexity of humanity and the certainty of eventual mortality. A year where I strengthened my focus on personal growth, ensuring future days would be better. Who knows, maybe it's because I turned 40, which to some is a milestone of midlife. Whether it's my mental health awakening, my midlife awakening, or perhaps the optimistic side of me finally coming to terms with some hard parts of life and figuring out how to work through them, instead of hiding from them. All I know is I feel so much more poignantly the thought that life is short. **I no longer want to accept living in a way that doesn't serve the life I envision. I don't want to live like I am dying, but rather I want to live fully.** Each day of our lives is such a gift, and just waiting to be unwrapped and appreciated.

I want to live each day as if it could be the best day of my life, and at a minimum, strive to make it better than the last. I don't want to take anyone or anything for granted. No day is guaranteed to lead to the next. The one guarantee and promise we each have is that we choose whether we see each day as a gift or a punishment. Do you continually look for joy and open yourself to positive moments, or do you seek sorrow and negativity? I don't remember being taught to see the good. That's the thing of life, we don't remember everything, but some things stick with us. Some perspectives in life challenge us. They challenge us to change the negative things we unknowingly learned. Once we can do that, those strong positive perspectives can shine through.

My hope is you'll never quit looking for the light at the end of the tunnel! It's always been there if you look for it, even on dark and scary days. I honestly believe you can find a silver lining in nearly every day if you choose to seek it. I may not be able to convince you to see the world the way I do, but I invite you to choose how you want your world to look. In the wise words of Yoda, "Do or do not, there is no try." Making choices can feel overwhelming or scary at times. That is our fear talking. What will hurt you more, in the long run, is not choosing the path you want your life to follow. If you just let the winds carry you, you leave your life in the control of others. Everyone's path will be a bit different, and you don't have to compete for first place. It's enough to just be a player in this game of life and enjoy your time in it. Every day you must show up swinging. Not every pitch will be good, and you won't necessarily hit a home run with each pitch that comes over the plate. Keep on swinging! Swing as if your life depends on it. Life is a treasure and it's up to each of us to not waste the gifts we've been given, and not waste time or energy on people and things that don't bring us good energy.

The person you will be tomorrow is determined by your actions today. So, choose the people, places, experiences, influences, and things you surround yourself with wisely. It matters! It always has and always will. Choose to live your life and each day of it in ways that align with the impact you want to make. In life, the only experiences to regret are the ones you don't take or leave yourself out of. As life plays out, we will all experience rough patches. Through each season of life, it's important to see the good and the unique opportunities. In tough times we often get the chance to dig deeper, reflect on life more, connect with our feelings more strongly, and through that, the opportunity to see what and who is important in life. The ones that show up on the good as well as the hard days. Those that share support whether we are smiling or crying. We can come to appreciate more the places that bring us joy and comfort. Let's hope we also take those opportunities to know what, where, and with whom we should be spending less time and energy.

Capture Beautiful Moments

If you're not taking those chances to experience all life has to offer, start! Be in the middle of it all. Be in the moment, share the words of love, and also take the pictures! Take the videos! Capture those moments in time with the people in your life. After losing both my grandma and my dad in a year and a half, both to aggressive, fast-growing forms of cancer, this is heartfelt advice I like to pass on. Capture those beautiful moments and memories, and not just family photos, friendships as well. Someday it may be the last photo or recording of someone's voice and mannerisms, and you'll be thankful for it.

What Are We Here For?

It's been a scary couple of years with all of the things that have impacted our world, but do you know why we've had this time? It's here to help us see that unless we have the courage to look back at the things that are hurting us, we will never see our way forward. Although life at times can feel scary or uncertain, we must remember we are here for a reason. We are all planted on Earth for a reason. We are here to grow and to help one another grow. Each of us has a unique passion and purpose and I want you to reach your full potential. We are here to believe in ourselves and others, to help build confidence, not break it down. Our words matter and we can each do our part to fill each other's lives with love and to help heal the hurts in our world, our communities, and our homes. If we choose to help spread the good as we each figure out our individual stories, the world will be a better place. As we each learn what our piece of the puzzle is, it's surely going to be a little messy. It won't always be pretty or perfect. Continue to take the next step. Keep looking for your inspiration, keep looking for the good and positive messages. The moment we quit looking for the good is the moment we utterly lose hope. That is the moment we quit trying to look for better ways to live our life. We each have a voice. Your story isn't over yet. We are all a tiny piece of the big puzzle. None of us can do this alone, it takes all of us. One person can have so much power. The power is inside you to make a difference. If you've been sitting on the sidelines, hiding in the shadows, or stuck on a loop—it's time to shake things up!

Perhaps you have closed your mind and heart over time. Open those doors, let the opportunities in. Stand up for what you believe in. Speak loud for what matters. It is not time to be small, it is not time to be quiet, it is not time to hide behind your fears. Speak up, even if your voice shakes— someone needs to hear it. Our future is bright, and we can do remarkable things. What are we waiting for? There is no time like the present. You have so much strength inside of you, and sometimes the greatest strength is being vulnerable and admitting when you've made a mistake. The world is full of mistakes and flaws. There's no reason to keep sweeping it under the rug. Time to shake it out, talk it out, and take a step forward. The right steps.

We All Have a Stone to Throw

Whether a stone or a starfish we all have something to throw into the game of life. Perhaps you've had a much different perspective on life, shaped in different ways. What I hope is that in reading this, may you be encouraged or challenged to consider a different perspective. Let's all quit faking it, let's discover and speak our truth and share it with others. Even if we don't believe the same things, we can challenge and help shape each other's views by broadening our understanding of each other. I hope this will speak to your heart in ways that will make a difference. A difference for good, a difference that will bring change. If we want to fix what's broken, if we want to ease the pain within ourselves and those around us, we must reach for happiness. We must encourage others and celebrate their success in finding their happiness. There is a place in our life for better things, and once we recognize what we truly value, we can take the next right action to get there.

Everyone is on a different point in this path, so always give yourself and others grace, compassion and please don't judge. We are not here to judge ourselves or others. Let's leave that to the judges with proper training. The first step is caring enough to make a difference and having confidence in yourself to be that difference. You've surely heard of the ripple effect; the impact of one small act. So, you see this is one big instruction manual about how you can make a ripple with your own stone. Toss it out there with love and kindness and try not to hurt anyone in the process. **Stop, look, listen— pause—consider your next right action to help create a better life for us all.**

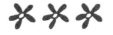

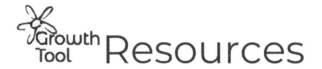

Growth Tool Resources

As I went on my journey in personal growth, I found a few resources helpful along the way. Perhaps they will help you discover the potential for happiness or be a part of what guides your path. A place to start...

Health & Wellness

Enter Into Calm, Christy Cowgill
Helpful Mind | Healthy Body | Healing Practices | Wellness
Proven program to refocus, restore, and recover from what ails or pains you through hypnosis www.enterintocalm.com

National Alliance on Mental Illness
NAMI, is the nation's largest grassroots mental health organization dedicated to building better lives for the millions of Americans affected by mental illness.

The NAMI HelpLine
can be reached Monday through Friday, 10 a.m. – 10 p.m., ET.
1-800-950-NAMI (6264) | info@nami.org
Text NAMI to 741-741 Connect with a trained crisis counselor to receive free, 24/7 crisis support via text message.

National Suicide Prevention Lifeline
Available 24 hours | 800-273-8255 | suicidepreventionlifeline.org

National Domestic Violence Hotline (24/7 guidance)
800-799-7233

Communication

Brené Brown
Vulnerability, Shame, and Leadership Researcher | Author | Speaker
brenebrown.com

Nonviolent Communication: A Language of Life: Life-Changing Tools for Healthy Relationships by Marshall B. Rosenberg PhD
Choice, Meaning and Connection | Connect Empathically | More Satisfying Relationships | Sharing of Resources

Thomas Gordon, Ph.D. The Gordon Model "I statement"
Communication Research | Conflict Resolution | Behavior Management | Active Listening
www.gordontraining.com/thomas-gordon/origins-of-the-gordon-model

Self-Discovery

Glennon Doyle
Mental Health Advocate | LGTBQ Cheerleader | Author | Speaker
momastery.com

Nicole Sachs, LCSW
Healing | Chronic Pain | Boundaries | Self-Love | Author | Speaker
www.TheCureForChronicPain.com

Vanessa and Xander Marin
Sex Therapist | Bedroom Communication Coach
vmtherapy.com/about-vanessa-marin

Here's How to Make a Vision Board for Manifestation
Oprah Daily
www.oprahdaily.com/life/a29959841/how-to-make-a-vision-board

Parenting With Humor

Kristina Kuzmic
Encouragement, Hope & Humor | Parenting | Mental Health Advocate | Life After Divorce
www.Kristinakuzmic.com

The Holderness Family
Parenting | Marriage | Real Life | Laughter | Mental Health Awareness
https://theholdernessfamily.com

Connect With Nature

Hike it Baby
Family Friendly | Community Support | Nature Advocate
www.HikeItBaby.com

Family Trail Guide
Family Friendly | Trails | Resource
trails.hikeitbaby.com/ftg-home

AllTrails
Trails | Resource | Hiking
www.alltrails.com

Marriage

Stephen Mitchell, Ph.D., and Erin Mitchell, MACP
Couples Counseling | Parenting | Communication Tools | Online Resources
createyourcouplestory.com | instagram.com/couples.counseling.for.parents

Marriage Continued...

Miracle Question, Solution Focused Therapy
A married therapist couple from Milwaukee, Steve de Shazer and Insoo Kim Berg are credited with the name and basic practice of SFT.
positivepsychology.com/miracle-question

Addiction, Recovery, Sober Life

SAMHSA
Substance Abuse and Mental Health Services Administration
1-877-SAMHSA-7
www.samhsa.gov

Decidedly Dry, Jessica Steitzer
Sober Culture | Healthy Living | Sober Mom Life
www.decidedlydry.com

Athletic Brewing
Non-Alcoholic Beer | Community Activism | Health & Wellness
Save 20% off your first online order with discount code: JillB20
www.AthleticBrewing.com

Tiffany Jenkins, Juggling the Jenkins
Mental Health Advocate | Comedian | Author | Addiction & Recovery
jugglingthejenkins.com

Dave Hollis
Health | Healing | Self Discovery | Life After Divorce |Sober Dad Life
www.mrdavehollis.com

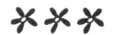

Acknowledgments

To the friends and family members that early on gave me words of support and encouragement as I continued to put one foot in front of the other on an unknown journey in writing and facing mental health struggles; it meant more to me than they may ever know. Big thanks to my husband who managed the household duties in the weeks and months as words poured from my heart to the keyboard and I was focused on other priorities to finish this book and keep up with my day job. I am grateful for my boys, Dean, Sam, and Peter who cheered me on with their excitement and were so interested that their mom was writing a book (*one in particular wanted to ensure his name was mentioned in the book, so I can now* ✔ *that off*).

So many thanks to my connections in the world of writing who gave sage advice and tips from their own experience to help me on this journey. I am so lucky to have been connected with my editor, Adam Swanson who so wonderfully polished my words to get them ready to publish and made me feel more confident in my writing. This chapter in my life would also not have been completed if not for the wonderful doctors and counselors who helped me learn to manage my mental and physical health to continue moving forward in life in a healthy, happy, and successful way.

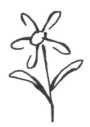

words to grow by

"Life is like an Etch a Sketch. You are in

control of the creation, so if you are not

happy with it, shake it up and try again."

About The Author

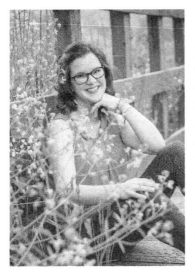

Jill (VanderZanden) Bilka

Jill is an outdoor loving, community supporting, craft beer drinking, business owner, and Mom of three that thrives on making a difference in her community. She is passionate about mental health awareness, advocating for local trails and ways to get people outside and active, as well as building community to help with overall wellness.

Jill thrives on making a difference in her community and the lives of others. She has a degree in Psychology, a working background in youth and family services as well as communication, and personal training in conflict resolution and leadership. She grew up the youngest of three girls in a small rural town in Oregon and is now raising her boys, Dean, Sam, and Peter in a small town in the heart of wine country.

Jill is a goal-oriented person that looks for success amidst struggles, opportunities in spite of obstacles, and a brighter purpose even when facing tough experiences. She enjoys working to help advance the mission of organizations and causes she is passionate about. Whether it's helping small businesses grow through effective communication and efficient operations or working to help advance the mission of organizations and causes, Jill cares deeply seeing programs, projects, and people succeed. In any situation, she works to connect the dots to help solve problems, find solutions, and provide resources. If Jill is not at home working or managing family life, you will likely find her out hiking or visiting a favorite local brewpub with friends.

Photo Credit: Sarah Morace Photography

Made in the USA
Monee, IL
19 June 2022

98271044R00085